The Montignac

DIET COOKBOOK

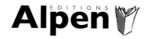

Alpen EDITIONS

Exclusive copyrights:
©Alpen Éditions
9, avenue Albert II
98000 Monaco
Tel: +377 97 77 62 10
Fax: +377 97 77 62 11
web: www.alpen.mc

Printed in Italy
ISBN: 978-2-35934-039-6

Starters
Photo credits: Bernard Radvaner
culinary stylist: Anne Sophie Lhomme
Thanks: Magasin Habitat

Fish
Photos credits: Eric Couderc
Culinary stylist: Laurence Fossati

Meats - Desserts
Photos credits: Anthony Lanneretonne
Culinary stylist: Carine Zurbach
Thanks: - Guy Degrenne and Tom Gueugnon
              - Shop "Le Faubourg", 3-11 rue Victor Cousin 06400 Cannes

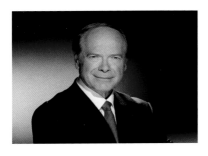

Introduction

The Montignac method*, created in France in 1986, was at first only geared to providing over-weight people with a way of losing weight easily and in a long-lasting way without imposing un-bearable dietary limits and restrictions. It then built its reputation on its efficacy. Word of mouth has always been its main reason for success.

From the first years after the book "Je mange, donc je maigris" (I Eat, Therefore I Lose Weight), one of the world's best-sellers in its field, was published, testimonies were not only about impres-sive, easy weight loss. The testimonies also mentioned beneficial side effects to health because of the changes made to eating habits when this method is applied.

This is how we discovered that following the Montignac method reduced cardiovascular risk fac-tors (cholesterol, triglycerides and hypertension, in particular) and also prevented and reduced the risk of developing type II diabetes.

When first few thousand readers of the book in France remarked that since traditional foods for the holidays there were allowed in the Montignac method (e.g. wine, champagne, foie gras paté and seafood), and France's traditional home-style dishes were allowed too (e.g. bean stew, pork and lentils, fish soup), this method of eating was a true combination of nutrition and gastronomy.

This is how a new concept was born: "Gastronomie Nutritionnelle®" (Nutritional Gastronomy), whose principles underlie all the "Montignac Recipes", which is particularly so for this book.

Cooking should be about pleasure first, and then also about pleasing others, those that we love in particular. But "Montignac cuisine" is, beyond tasting good, being certain that the meal we pre-pare is extremely healthy.

I wish you the very best in using the recipes in this book.

Michel Montignac.

* To find out more about the Montignac method, visit: www.montignac.com

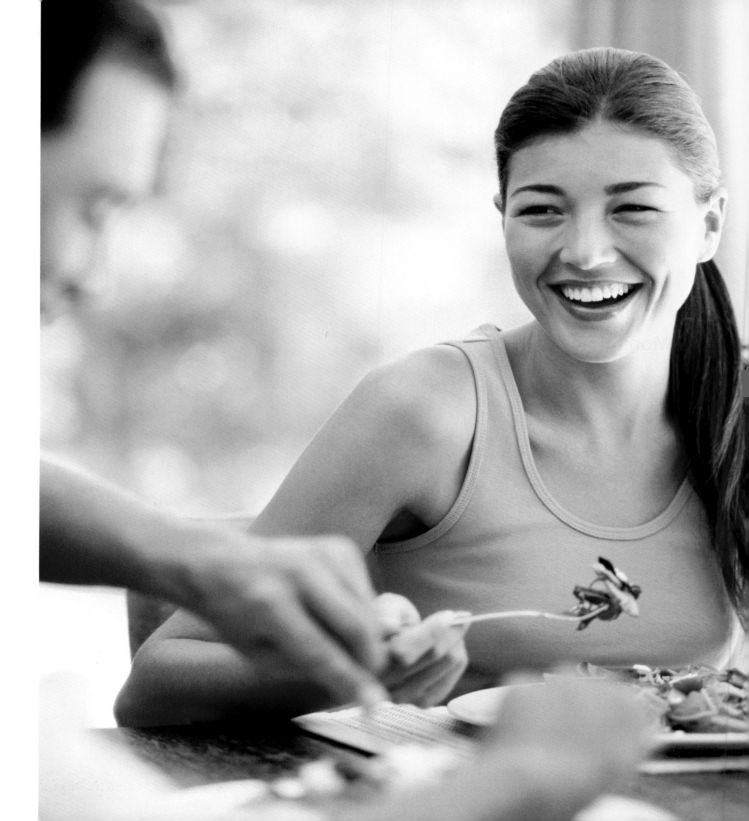

Contents

The failure of
the low calorie diet

Over the last century, obesity has risen by a factor of about eight in western countries. The worst problem is in the United States, where 35% of the population is obese today, but this scourge is not only affecting industrialized countries now.

In 1997 the World Health Organization (WHO) raised the alarm when it decreed that the whole world was now affected by what had become at that time an epidemic.

This phenomenon is without precedent in human history, so let's try to understand some of its causes. By discovering the real reasons for it we also understand why, even if we are not obese, we tend to gain weight so easily nowadays.

If we understand it then we discover how we can not only lose our excess weight, but how we stay at our ideal weight forever by using a few basic principles that still allow us to eat normal amounts, including festive foods such as chocolate, the French favorite foie gras paté, and wine.

The American paradox

In the 1930's, when the obesity level in the United States reached 8%, a number of doctors decided to try to determine the phenomenon's causes. The United States was already producing more food than it needed. Mechanization and comfort becoming more general reduced the population's energy output, and a group of scientists reached the following conclusion very quickly.

If Americans become fatter and fatter, it is for two reasons: firstly they eat too much, and secondly they do not use enough energy.

This is how the principle of "energy balance" was officially defined, whereby, if a person wanted to lose weight, he had to eat less (follow a low-calorie diet) and exercise more. Since the 1940's Americans who were convinced that this argument made sense have been applying this nutritional theory of energy balance strictly.

A food's calorie counts became such an obsession that almost 80% of Americans eat low-calorie products today. A dread of fat has almost become paranoia. As well as this, Americans consume the highest amounts of artificial sugars (synthetic sweeteners) and spend the most time exercising.

The US holding the honors for the world's obesity levels should make us seriously doubt how effective this routine is. Obsessive reduction of

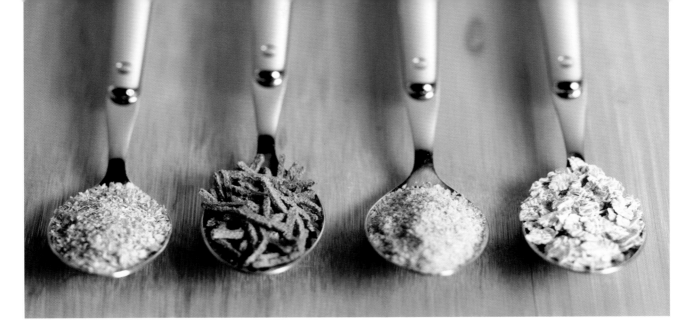

Phase II : stabilization and prevention phase

Carbohydrates are still selected according to their glycemic index (GI) in Phase II, but the selection is wider than in Phase I.

In this Phase the choices can even be refined by using a new concept, which is a meal's **glycemic balance.** This means that all carbohydrates can be eaten under some conditions, even those with high glycemic indexes.

A world-famous method

The Montignac method is known all over the world (18 million books sold in 45 countries and translated into 26 languages) because it is considered as being the best alternative to the obviously unsuccessful low-calorie diet.

Its legitimacy stems from the combined wisdom of several hundred scientific studies published in the last twenty years and also from the experience and testimonies of tens of thousands of people who have tried it and succeeded in losing weight, including doctors who prescribe it.

At the end of the 1980's Michel Montignac was the first person to propose using the concept of glycemic index for weight loss. He was followed (and copied) by many opinion leaders in the health field.

From this he has become one of its specialists, on both mastery of the concept and how to apply it practically to reduce and prevent metabolic diseases such as obesity, diabetes and cardiovascular disease.

To find out more about the Montignac method and to see the many books published in this area, visit site www.montignac.com

Montignac cuisine
in detail

This recipe book is obviously designed around the principles of the Montignac method. Accordingly, none of the recipes contains bad carbohydrates such as sugar, white flour, potatoes, corn or white or sticky rice.

A number of substitution techniques are proposed to replace some traditional cooking techniques, such as binding sauces or using flour in cakes.

Many replacement possibilities are suggested for the pasta, potatoes and rice that are too often present in the usual "food landscape". We don't need these when we have other excellent starches (lentils, beans, peas and others) and a range of vegetables so varied that everyone will find something to enjoy.

Most of the recipes in this book are inspired by Provencal, or more generally, Mediterranean cuisine. There are three reasons for this.

• First, my personal taste developed over eight years when I was fortunate enough to live in the south-east of France.

• Second, because it has now been officially recognized by all the international health bodies that the Mediterranean diet is the best in the world,

in particular that it is the one that best prevents cardiovascular disease.

• Last and especially because Provencal-type recipes are always very simple to make.

The culinary options for the Montignac method

Some of the options might surprise professional cooks, even cause them to shrug their shoulders in wonder.

• **Regarding fat**

Butter is excluded from any Montignac recipe on principle because it is a food that decomposes when cooked and becomes rather indigestible, even carcinogenic.

To replace it, you can use almost unlimited **olive oil and goose or duck fat**. Goose and duck fat have the same molecular structure as olive oil (oleic acid).

Whenever a recipe contains cream or sour cream, you should use a reduced-fat alternative or replace it with soy cream.

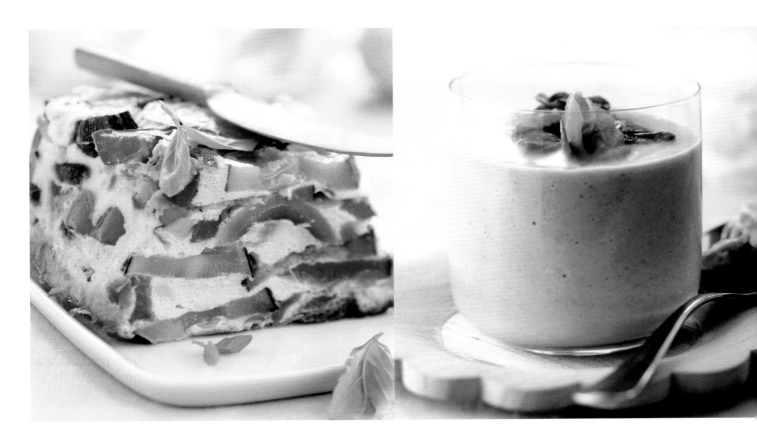

• Regarding cooking

One of the options that I suggest in the book is low-temperature cooking. Whether we are cooking onions in a pan, or vegetables, fish, seafood or even some meats (poultry in particular), there is no need for high heat that caramelizes the food excessively (or even burns it).

Too much cooking destroys the food's molecular structure, which makes it hard to digest and even harmful to health.

• Desserts are a revolution

I was once on a television program along with one of France's most famous pastry chefs. The journalist asked me what was special about a Montignac dessert. I replied: "It's a dessert that contains no sugar, butter, or flour!"
The pastry chef burst out laughing! He declared ironically: "But sugar, butter and flour are the basis of pastry and desserts. What's left in a Montignac dessert?"

I will leave you to discover that for yourself.

The characteristics of
Montignac desserts

Various substitution techniques are proposed to replace traditional dessert making practices.

The main principles of Montignac desserts

First of all these are characterized by their lack of the main ingredients used in traditional desserts. Montignac desserts do not contain flour, sugar or butter.

No flour

Traditional desserts are almost all made from flour. White flour, naturally. Yet this product is excluded in the Montignac method since its glycemic index is very high (85).

In addition, either the flour is completely absent from the recipe, which actually makes it original, or it is replaced with another ingredient with a low glycemic index. This is especially true when you make a *fond de succès* (sponge cake). In particular, the flour is replaced by almond powder.

As an exception, some desserts may be made with whole-wheat flour as long as it is real. As its GI is higher than 35, an attempt will be made to add ingredients to the recipe that can help lower the glycemic outcome (GO) of the cake: apple, pectin or even agar-agar or carob.

No sugar

Traditional desserts are all, without exception, made with sugar. You know that sugar with its high glycemic index (70) is banned in the Montignac method. So, when necessary, we'll suggest sweetening the Montignac desserts with fructose. Fructose has the advantage of being a real sugar and thus a natural product. But its main quality is that it has a very low glycemic index (20). It is also just as easy to work with as sugar since its weight is almost identical. The only thing you need to remember is that fructose has a sweetening potential almost two times that of sugar. So two times less needs to be used.

No butter

Butter has various problems. The main one is that it is a saturated fat. What you need to know is that saturated fatty acids are the ones most likely to store fat reserves in the body. In other words, butter like meat fat or cold cuts are a factor for gaining weight.

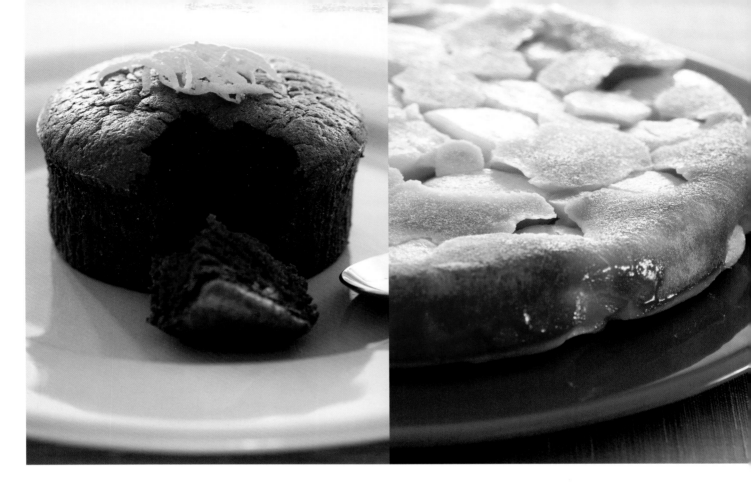

Another problem with butter, again like all saturated fats, is that it is a cardiovascular risk factor. This is why people who have high cholesterol should avoid it. In addition, you should also know that cooked butter is very bad for your health. At 100°C, its short chain fatty acids are destroyed and become indigestible, since it is difficult for digestive enzymes to break them down. But starting from 120°, butter completely spoils. It also forms acrolein, recognized as a carcinogen.

This is why butter is not included in the Montignac dessert recipes. When needed, which is not always the case, it will be replaced by olive oil or goose fat, monounsaturated fatty acids, which are not just very beneficial for your health, but also have the advantage of not spoiling with cooking time.

And you'll see that from a taste standpoint, this replacement is just amazing.

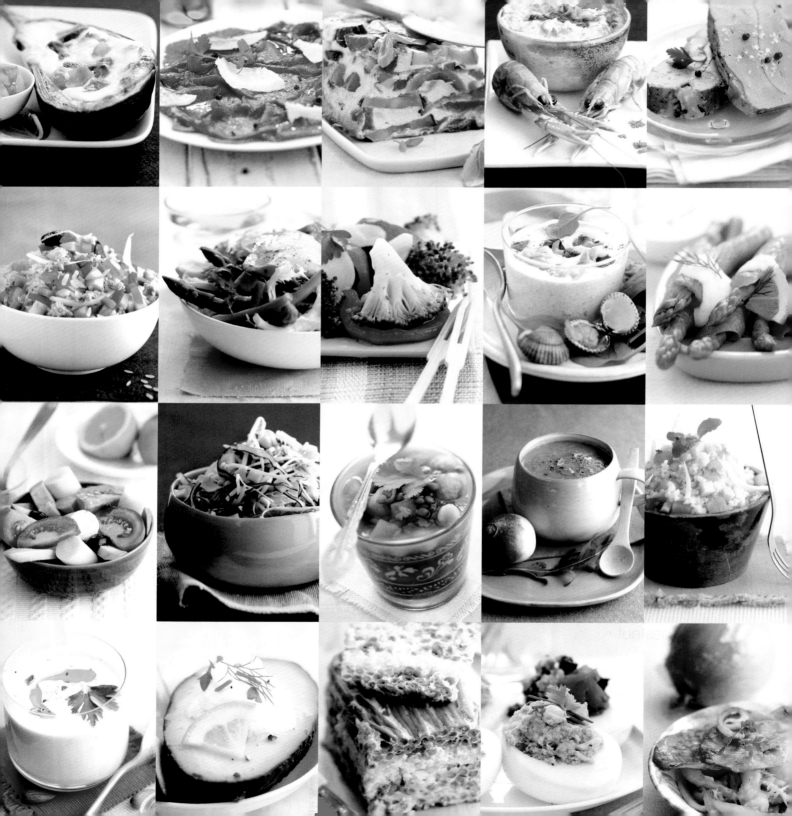

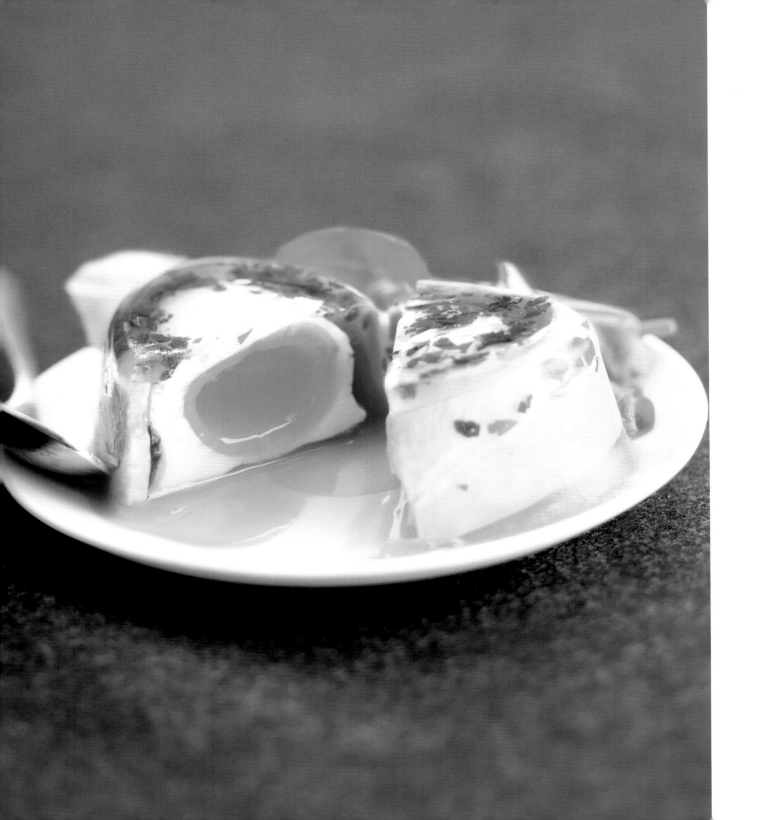

Aubergines stuffed with tomato and mozzarella cheese

Serves 4

Preparation: 10 minutes
Cooking time: 40 minutes

- 2 aubergines
- 2 tomatoes
- 7oz (200 g) mozzarella
- 4 anchovy fillets
- 1/2 teaspoon oregano
- Salt, pepper

- Cut the aubergines in two and wrap in kitchen foil.
- Bake in a moderate oven at 190°C (375°F, gas mark 5) for 30 minutes.
- Plunge the tomatoes into boiling water for 30 seconds, skin and remove the seeds. Dice the f1esh.
- Arrange the aubergines in an oven-proof dish. Fill them with the chopped tomatoes and season with salt and pepper. Cover with strips of mozzarella and an anchovy fillet.
- Finally, add the oregano. Place in the oven at 250°C (500°F, gas mark 9) for 7-10 minutes until the cheese is melted and golden brown. Serve immediately.

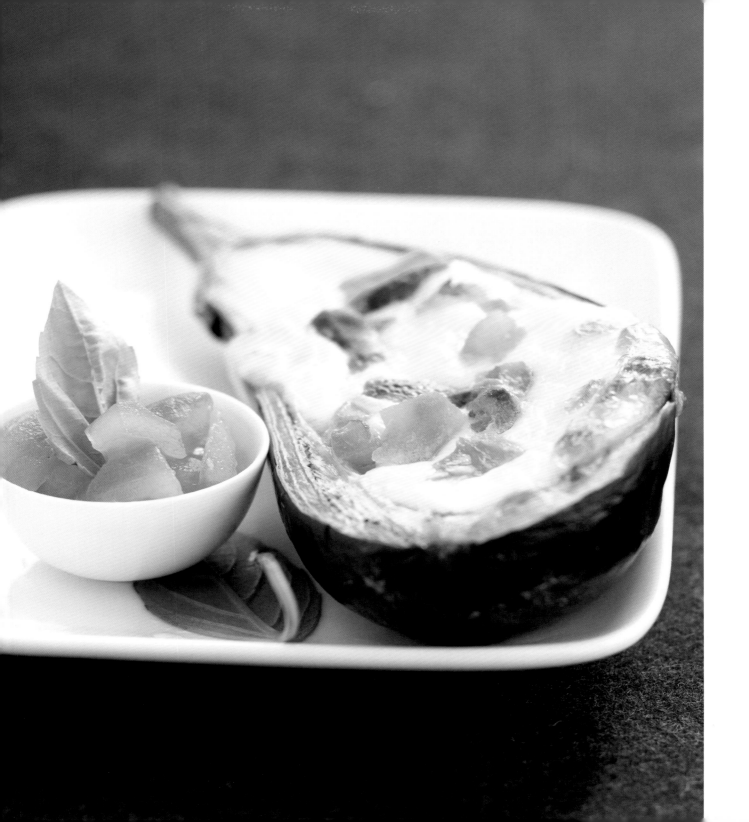

Avocados with fromage frais

Serves 6

Preparation: 20 minutes

- 3 large ripe avocados
- 7oz (200 g) fromage frais (not low fat)
- 1 full-fat natural yogurt
- 1 small clove garlic
- 1 small bunch parsley
- 1 small bunch chives
- 1 small bunch dill
- 2 egg whites
- Lemon juice
- Olive oil
- Salt, pepper

- Cut the avocados in half and remove the stones. Combine the yogurt with the fromage frais, the crushed garlic and the chopped herbs.
- Season with a dash of lemon juice, olive oil, salt and pepper.
- Beat the egg whites until stiff and fold gently into the mixture to obtain a mousse-like consistency.
- Spoon this onto the avocados and serve chilled.

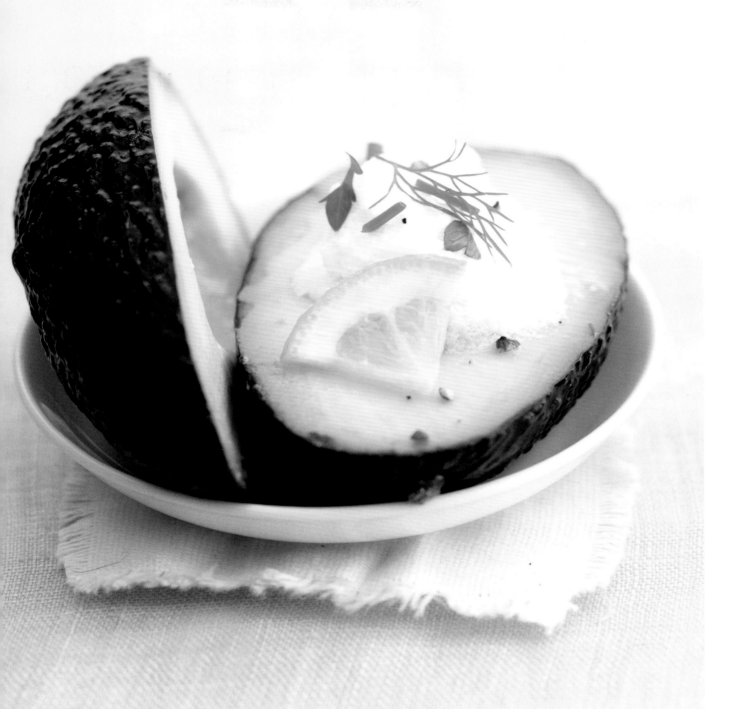

Beef Carpaccio

Serves 4

Preparation: 10 minutes

- 11oz (300g) Carpaccio
- Olive oil
- Granular sea salt
- Freshly ground pepper
- Herbes de Provence

- Carpaccio is prepared from raw beef, either top-rump or fillet, which has been finely sliced on a butcher's slicing machine. Ask your butcher to interleave with greaseproof paper to prevent the slices sticking together. If preparing the meat at home, to make it and easier to handle freeze briefly before slicing.
- Arrange the Carpaccio on large plates.
- Brush with olive oil.
- Sprinkle lightly with the Herbes de Provence, coarse sea salt and pepper from the pepper mill.
- Allow to stand and marinate for 10 to 15 minutes before serving.

Variation:
Replace Herbes de Provence with flakes of Parmesan cheese thinly pared with a potato peeler.

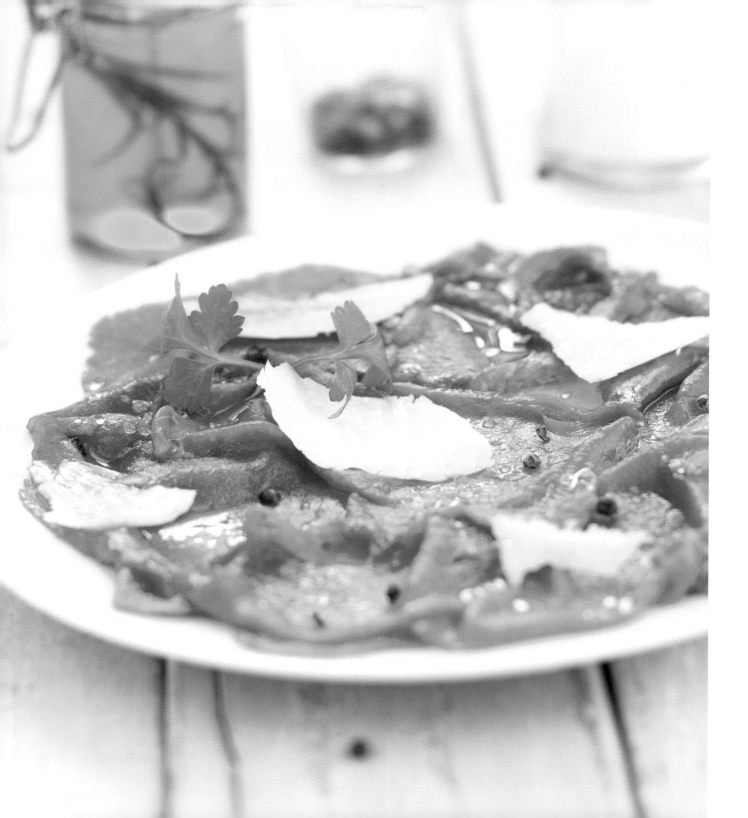

Cucumber with fennel, mint and yogurt dressing

Serves 6

Preparation: 30 minutes

- 3 cucumbers
- 3 natural yogurts
- 1 teaspoon chopped fresh fennel
- 3 tablespoons olive oil
- 1 teaspoon chopped fresh mint
- 1 teaspoon salt
- 2 tablespoons wine vinegar
- 2 cloves garlic

- Peel the cucumbers, slice them in two, remove the pips and seeds and chop into small pieces. Cover with rough salt to draw out the liquid and leave for 15 minutes.
- Crush the garlic and place in a bowl with the vinegar. Leave to marinate for 10 minutes. Then, in another bowl, mix the yogurt, olive oil and fennel.
- Pour the vinegar through a fine sieve and add to the yogurt mixture.
- Drain the cucumbers thoroughly, rinse, and dry.
- Serve the cucumber with the yogurt dressing, sprinkled with chopped mint.

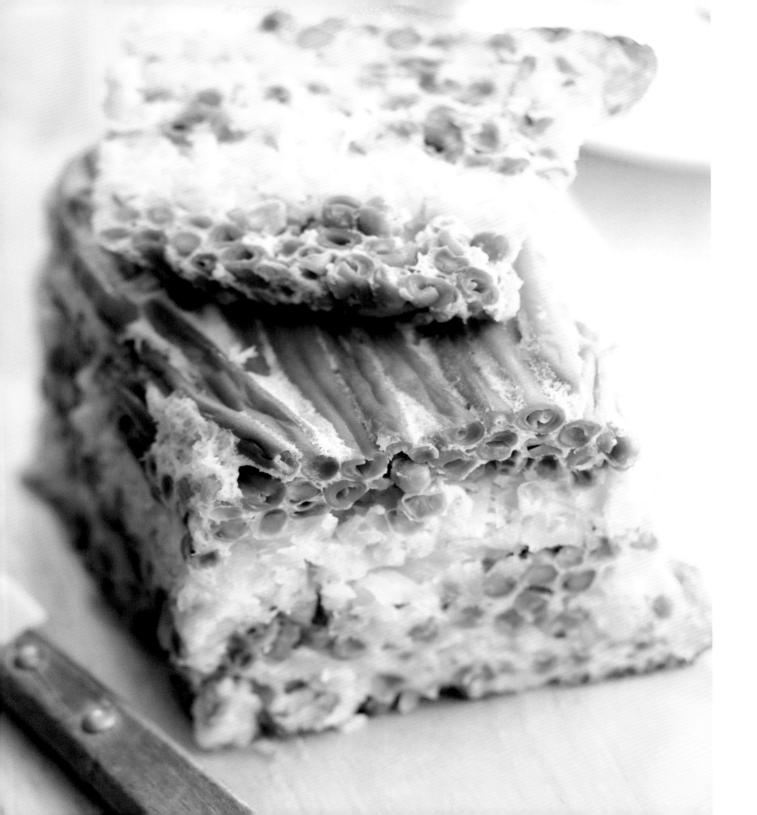

Cheese and ginger mould

Serves 6

Preparation: 18 minutes
Cooking time: 25 minutes

- 4oz (100 g) ginger (diced)
- 9oz (250 g) fromage frais with 15% fat
- 3 eggs
- 4 leaves of gelatine (or the equivalent of agar-agar)
- 2oz (60 ml) full cream milk
- Salt, pepper

- The day before, immerse the ginger in water.
- Immerse the leaves of gelatine in cold water.
- Beat the egg yolks and add the fromage frais.
- Beat the egg whites until they are stiff and add to the mixture.
- Heat the milk. Drain the leaves of gelatine and then, add to the milk.
- Add this liquid to the mixture and the, add the ginger drained. Mix delicately. Season with salt and pepper.
- Pour the mixture into a mould and cook in a hot oven at 220 °C (440 °F, gas mark 7) for 25 minutes. Serve hot or cold.

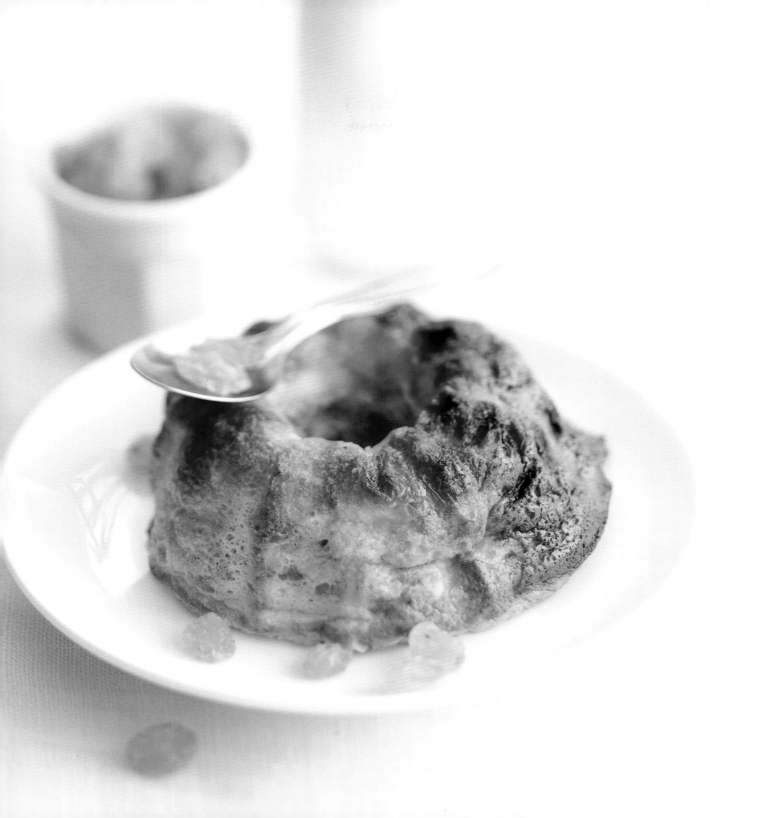

Turbot mould with watercress coulis Serves 4

Preparation: 15 minutes
Cooking time: 1 hour 15 minutes

- 1lb (500 g) turbot fillets
- 8 scampi (Dublin Bay prawns, langoustines)
- 1 bunch watercress
- 7fl oz (20 cl) low fat whipping cream
- 1 pint (50 cl) low fat crème fraiche
- 2 eggs and 2 egg whites
- 1 bouquet garni
- 1 court bouillon
- Olive oil
- Salt, pepper

- Cook turbot fillets in a court-bouillon with the bouquet garni, salt and pepper for 20 minutes and then, drain the fish.
- Cook the scampi for 2 minutes in boiling salted water and shell them.
- Pour the turbot fillets through the blender, beat the eggs and add to the fish.
- Add the crème fraiche. Season with salt and pepper.
- Beat the egg whites until stiff and fold gently into the mixture to obtain a mousse-like consistency.
- Oil 4 individual moulds and pour 1 or 2 scampi in. Then pour the mixture and cover with a sheet of kitchen foil. Cook in a bain-marie in medium over at 160/180 °C (320/360 °F, gas mark 4-5) for 20 minutes.
- Wash the watercress and blanch for 5 minutes in boiling salted water. Drain, pour through the blender and sieve. Before serving, add the whipping cream to the watercress and heat gently without boiling. Adjust the seasoning.
- Turn out turbot moulds and serve with the watercress coulis.

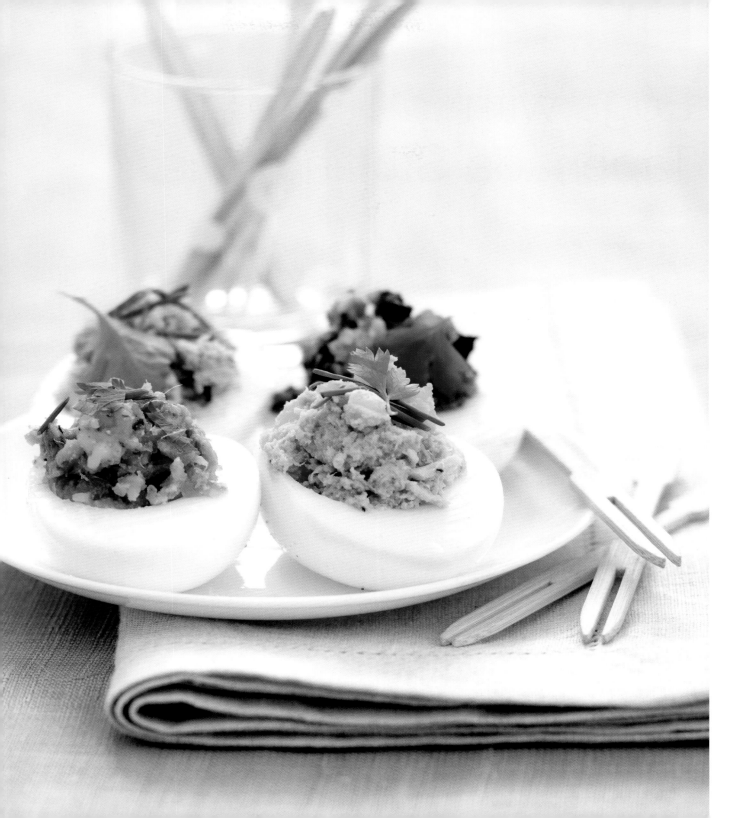

Eggs with Tapenade Stuffing Serves 4

Preparation: 15 minutes
Cooking time: 10 minutes

- 6 eggs
- 1 small jar (1 1/2 oz or 40 g) tapenade
- 1 tablespoon olive oil
- Lettuce leaves
- Brunch of parsley

- Boil the eggs for 10 minutes until hard. Cool in cold water.
- Remove the shell and cut lengthways into two.
- Scoop out the yolk with a small spoon and place the whites on a serving dish covered with lettuce leaves.
- Crush the yolks with a fork and mix with the tapenade and olive oil, to make a smooth paste.
- Using the small spoon, fill the whites with the mixture.
- Sprinkle freshly chopped parsley over the eggs and serve.

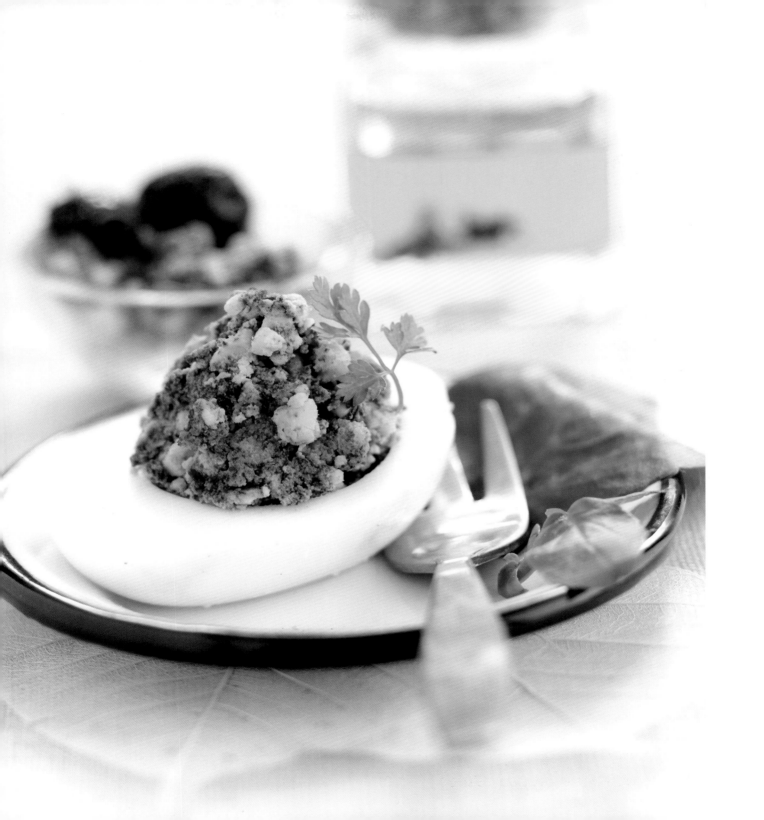

Cheese and Onion Rösti with Bacon

Serves 4

Preparation: 15 minutes
Cooking time: 20 minutes

- 8 onion
- 14oz (400g) grated Gruyère cheese
- 8 slices bacon
- Olive oil
- Freshly ground pepper

- Peel and chap the onions.
- Take a large pan, add olive oil and the chopped onions, and heat gently to a golden brown. Season with freshly ground pepper.
- Degrease the onion by turning out into absorbent kitchen paper.
- On individual oven-proof dishes make beds of onions and cover each portion with 100g (3 ½ oz) of Gruyère cheese.
- Cover each bed with 2 slices of bacon and place 10 cm (4in) below the grill in a very hot oven, preheated at 240°C (480°F, gas mark 10).
- Take out and serve when the cheese is slightly browned.

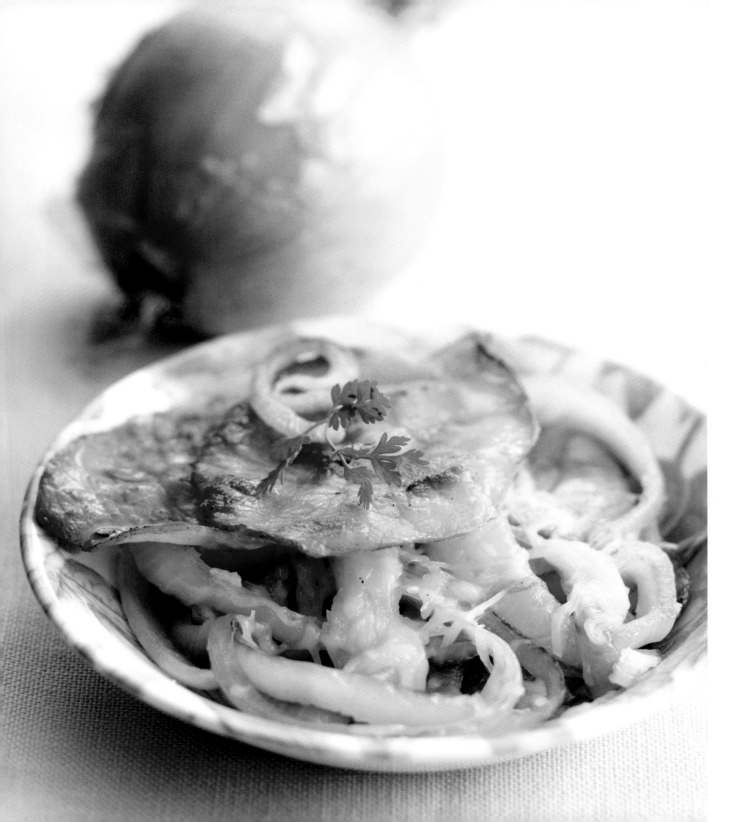

Avocado Pâté
with prawns   Serves 4

Preparation: 15 minutes
Cooking time: 2 minutes
Refrigeration 6 hours

- 5 ripe avocados
- 9oz (250 g) prawns – pealed
- 2 lemons
- 1/2oz (12 g) agar-agar
- 3 tablespoons Montbazillac (white semi-sweet wine from the Bergerac)
- 1 teaspoon ground green peppercorns
- Salt, Cayenne pepper

- Pat the prawns dry.
- Mix the avocado flesh with the lemon juice and the ground green peppercorns.
- Dissolve the agar-agar in the Montbazillac by warming gently.
- Season with salt and Cayenne pepper and mix well.
- Pour into a mould and pat down well.
- Place in the fridge for at least 6 hours.
- Serve on a bed of lettuce with a light mayonnaise.

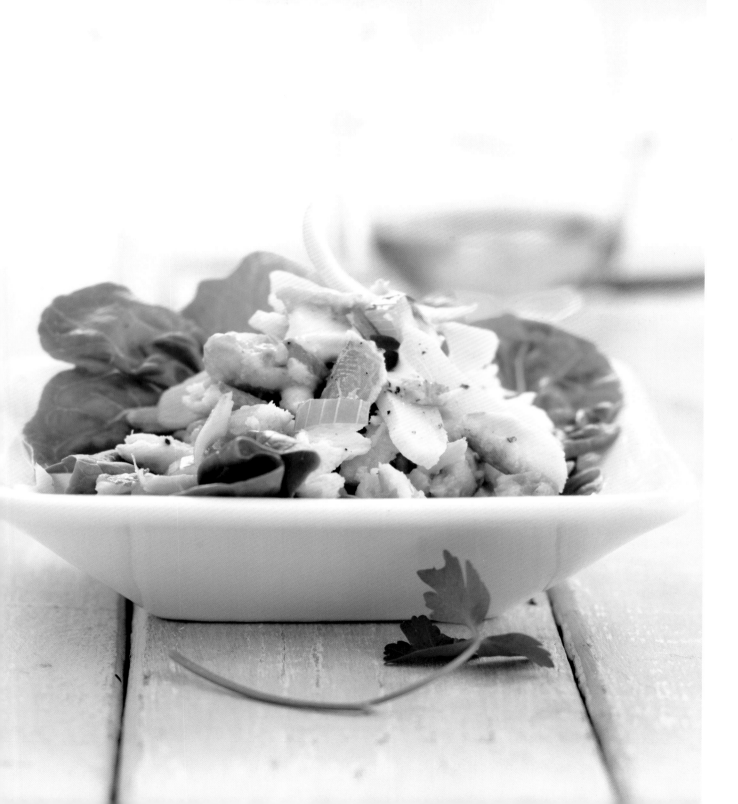

Foie gras with asparagus
and artichoke salad

Serves 6

Preparation: 40 minutes
Cooking time: 30 minutes

- 1lb (500 g) small fresh French beans
- 1lb (500 g) green asparagus
- 2 raw artichoke bases
- 1 head frisée lettuce
- 6 slices foie gras (3oz - 70 g each)
- Leman juice

For the vinaigrette:
- 6 tablespoons sunflower oil
- 2 tablespoons sherry vinegar
- Salt, pepper

- Dip the artichoke bases in lemon juice, cook in boiling water and cut into pieces.
- Cook the French beans in salted boiling water, making sure they remain firm, and drain. Trim and cook the asparagus in the same way and drain. Allow all the vegetables to cool and mix them together. Wash and spin the salad
- Prepare a vinaigrette from 6 tablespoons of sunflower oil, 2 tablespoons of sherry vinegar, salt and pepper.
- Pour the dressing over the vegetables.
- On each plate place two or three good-sized lettuce leaves, some of the vegetable salad and a slice of foie gras. Serve at once.

Suggestion :
It is possible to use tinned artichoke bases, in which case they will not require cooking.

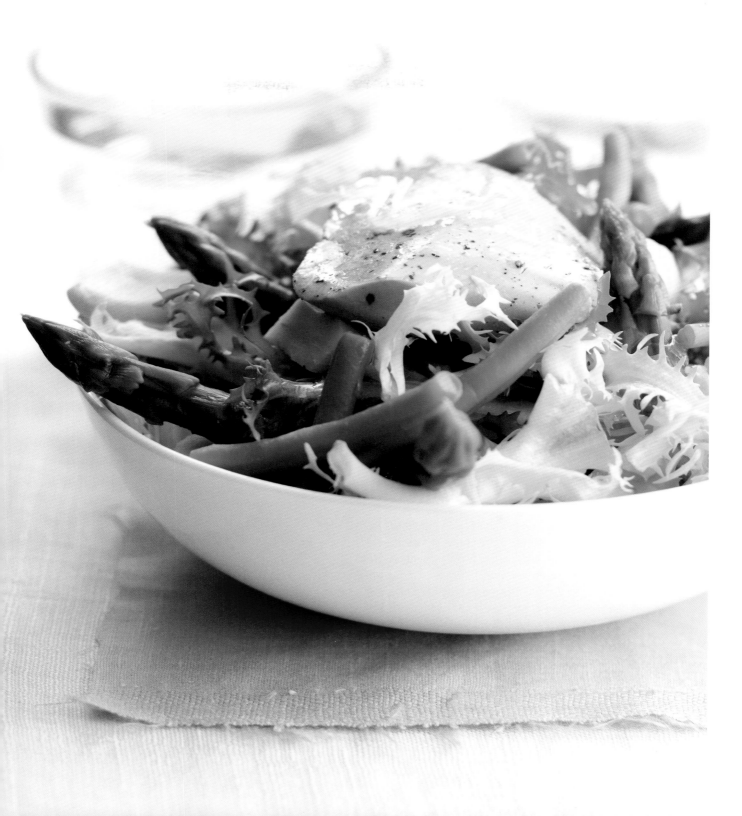

Scallops with an artichoke, pistachio, and chestnut salad

Serves 4

Preparation: 30 minutes

- 1 head frisée lettuce
- 1 Batavia lettuce
- 2oz (50 g) dried pistachios
- 4 cooked artichoke bases
- 12oz (350 g) scallops cooked and shelled
- 7oz (200 g) chestnuts in water
- 9oz (250 g) vinaigrette (olive oil and vinegar)
- Tarragon, chives
- Salt, pepper

- Wash and spin the lettuces. Chop the pistachios and add them to the vinaigrette. Cut the artichoke bases into strips and dip them in the vinaigrette.
- Slice the scallops, season with salt, pepper and the vinaigrette and marinade for 15 minutes.
- Mix the lettuce with the vinaigrette and the finely chopped chestnuts.
- Arrange the scallops on top and decorate with the artichoke, tarragon and chopped chives.

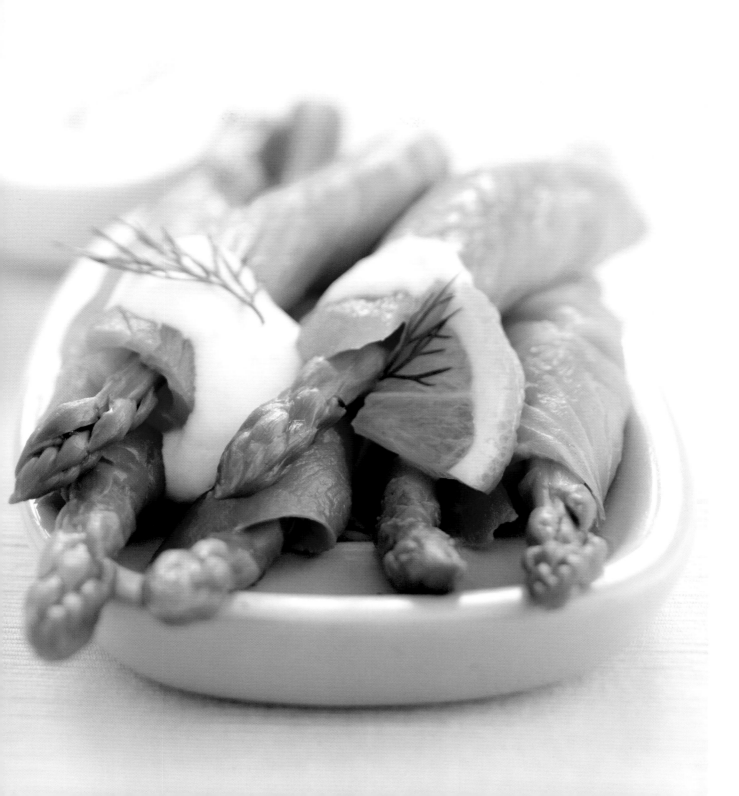

Avocado and
red pepper salad Serves 4

Preparation: 10 minutes
Cooking time: 15 à 20 minutes

- 2 ripe avocados
- 2 red peppers
- 4 Belgian endives
- Some leaves of mesclun
- 2 tablespoons chopped parsley
- 20 stoned black olives
- Provençale vinaigrette (olive oil, garlic, herbes de Provence…)
- Lemon

- Put the red peppers into a pre-heated oven at 200°C (400°F, gas mark 5) or steamer until bliste-red. Cool and peel. Cut into thin strips.
- Peel the avocados, cut into pieces, and dip in lemon juice to avoid discoloration.
- Shred finely the olives.
- Cut Belgian endives into thick slices.
- On individual plates, arrange the salad with avocados, endives, and red pepper on the top.
- Put the vinaigrette over the dish and sprinkle with chopped parsley and olives.

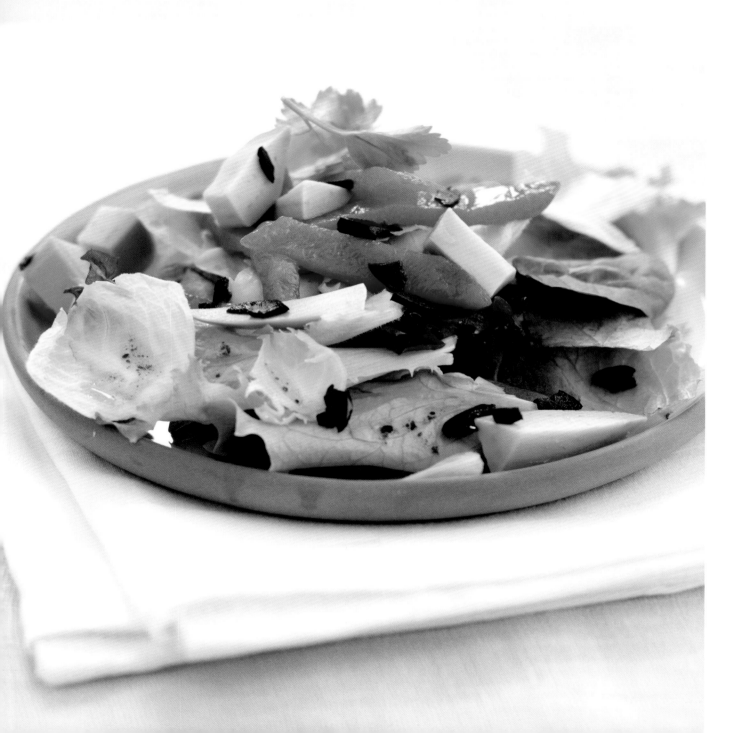

Salad of spinach and cockles   Serves 6

Preparation: 30 minutes
Cooking time: 10 minutes

- 3 lb (1,4 kg) cockles
- 1¾ lb (800 g) spinach
- 7oz (200 ml) white wine
- 7oz (200 g) low-fat whipping cream
- 3 tomatoes
- 1 shallot
- Nutmeg
- Sherry vinegar
- Chives
- Paprika

- Rinse the cockles several times and dry them. Heat the white wine with the shallot and add the cockles, on a high heat, so that they open up. Remove from their shells.
- Trim and wash the spinach. Cook half of it in boiling salted water for 5 minutes. Drain and put through the blender, with the salt, pepper, nutmeg and sherry vinegar.
- Whip the cream until stiff (like Chantilly), then fold it into the spinach mixture. Chop the remainder of the raw spinach finely
- Place the spinach mixture in the centre of the plate, add the cockles, and surround with the raw spinach.
- Garnish with tomato quarters and sprinkle with chives and paprika. Serve immediately.

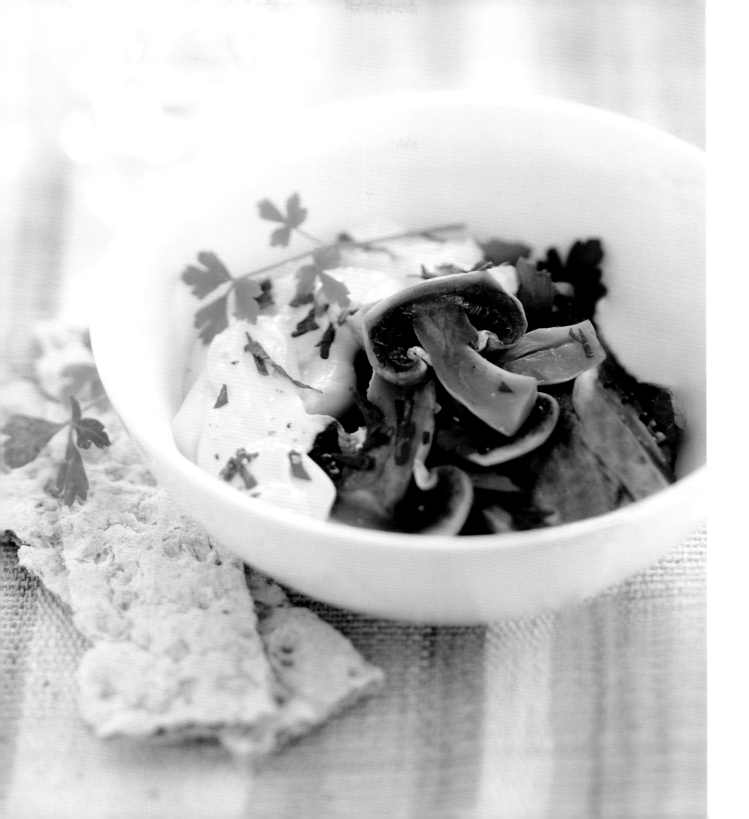

White cabbage
salad with bacon Serves 8

Preparation: 30 minutes
Cooking time: 5 minutes

- 1 large hard white cabbage
- 14oz (400 g) smoked streaky bacon (in a piece not rashers)
- 5 hard-boiled eggs
- Chopped parsley
- Vinaigrette (olive oil, vinegar, mustard, salt, pepper)

- Remove the outside leaves and wash the cabbage under running water. Dry with a cloth or absorbent kitchen paper.
- Halve or quarter the cabbage and shred fine1y, using a sharp knife.
- Cut the hard-boiled eggs in half and remove the yolks. Make the yolks into a "mimosa", using a "moulinette" if you have one.
- Cut the whites into little cubes or thin strips.
- Dice the bacon, discarding the ends if they are very fat. Fry very gently in a non-stick pan, greased with a little olive oil.
- Make a classic vinaigrette from olive oil, mustard, vinegar, salt and pepper.
- Transfer the cabbage first to the serving dish or individual plates. Scatter the egg whites over it and then, sprinkle with the "mimosa" of egg yolks and the chopped parsley.
- Season with the vinaigrette.
- Add the hot diced bacon at the last minute.

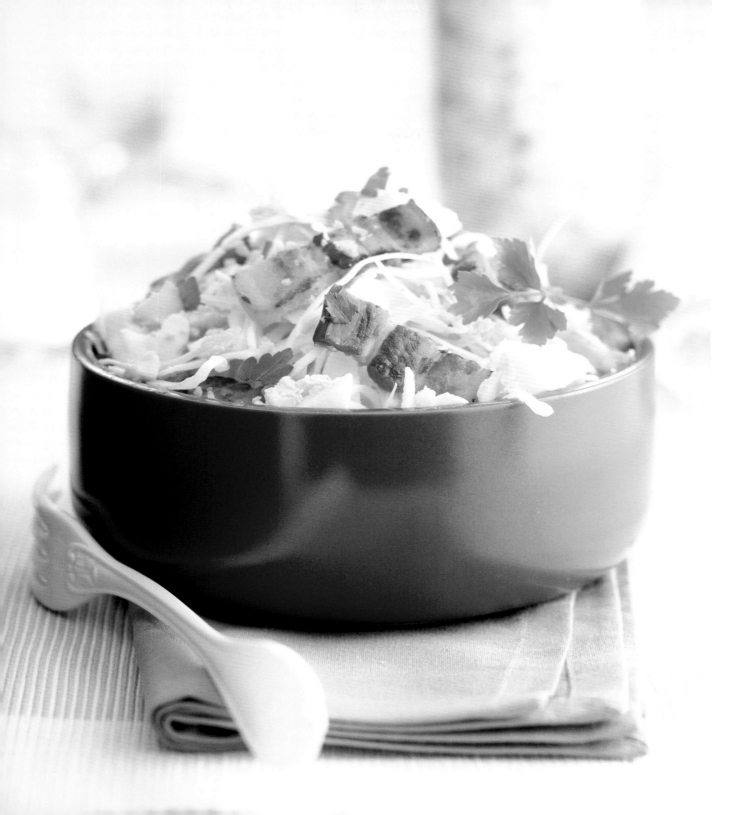

Red Cabbage
Salad with Walnuts Serves 5

Preparation: 15 minutes

- 1 small red cabbage
- 1 onion – thinly sliced
- 2 tablespoons olive oil
- 2 tablespoons red wine vinegar
- 2 teaspoons walnut oil
- 2 teaspoons mustard
- 2oz (50 g) walnuts very coarsely chopped
- Salt, freshly ground pepper

- Remove the outside leaves of the cabbage. Quarter and slice thinly.
- Peel the onion and cut into thin slices. Ensure the slices break up into rings.
- Prepare the vinaigrette: dissolve the salt and mustard in the vinegar. Add the pepper, olive oil and walnut oil. Mix well.
- Put the cabbage in a bowl, add the vinaigrette and walnuts.

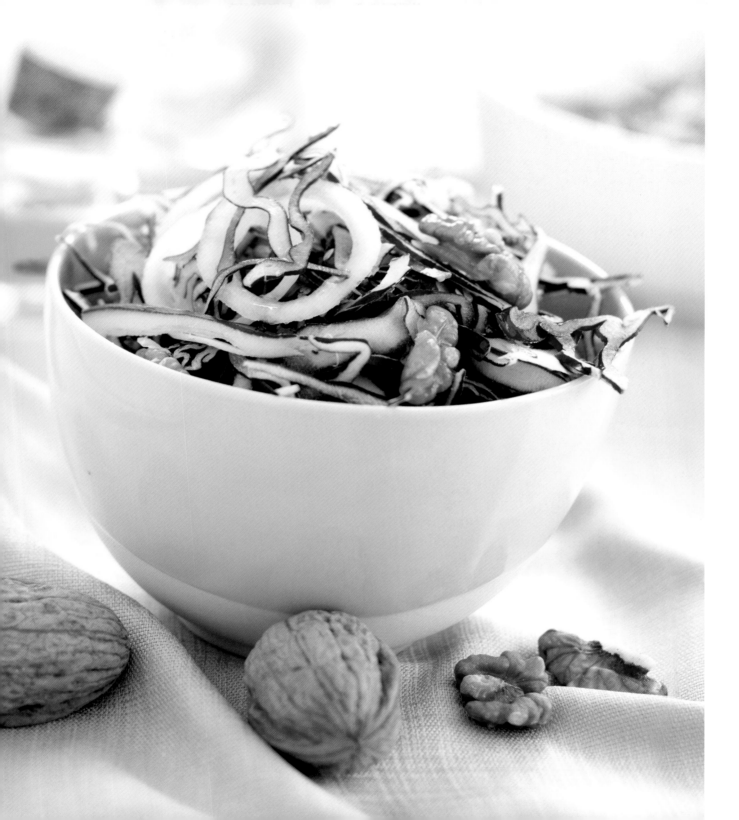

Scallops served with sauerkraut and asparagus

Serves 4

Preparation: 10 minutes
Cooking time: 7 minutes

- 21oz (600 g) raw sauerkraut
- 12 asparagus tips
- 8 raw scallops
- Juice of 1 lemon
- 3 tablespoons olive ail
- Chervil, salt, pepper

- Marinade the sauerkraut in the lemon juice, salt, pepper and olive ail. Steam the asparagus tips for 7 minutes or cook in salted boiling water for 5 minutes.
- Cut each of the scallops in half. Cook in a frying-pan over a high heat for 1 minute each side.
- Season with salt and pepper.
- Place the sauerkraut on individual plates and arrange the scallops and asparagus on top.
- To serve, decorate with chervil.

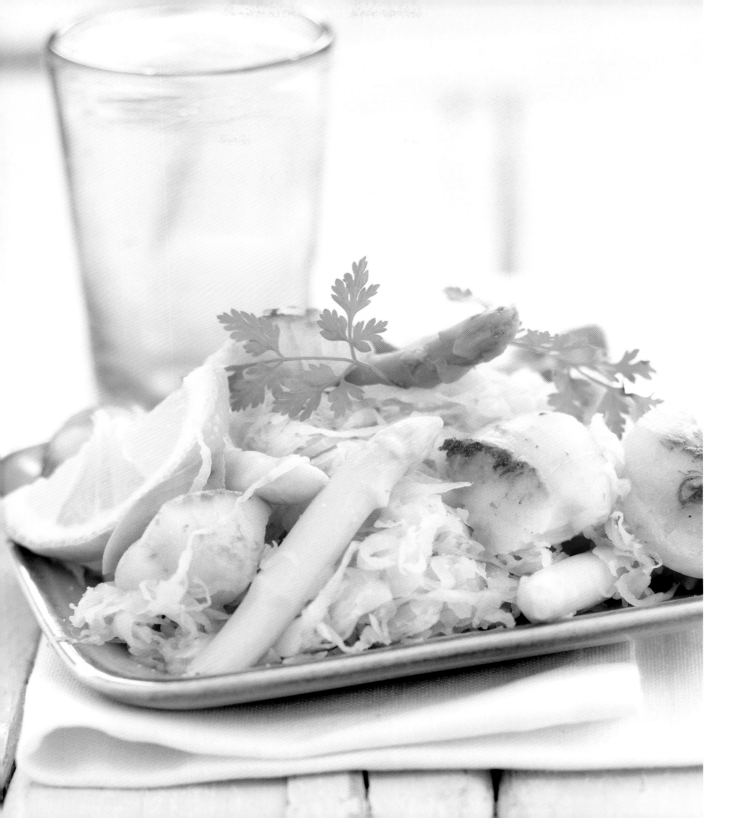

Watercress
and Bacon Salad Serves 4

Preparation: 15 minutes
Cooking time: 12 minutes

- 12oz (350 g) watercress
- 4oz (100 g) diced streaky bacon
- ½ glass sherry vinegar
- Olive oil

- Dice the streaky bacon. Blanch for 4 minutes in boiling unsalted water. Drain.
- Fry the diced streaky bacon in a non-stick pan over a low heat until the fat has melted.
- Sort and wash the watercress. Drain and transfer to a large bowl.
- Throw away the melted bacon fat and deglaze the pan with the sherry vinegar. Turn the diced bacon and deglazing over the watercress. Dribble olive oil over the top.
- Toss the salad and serve.

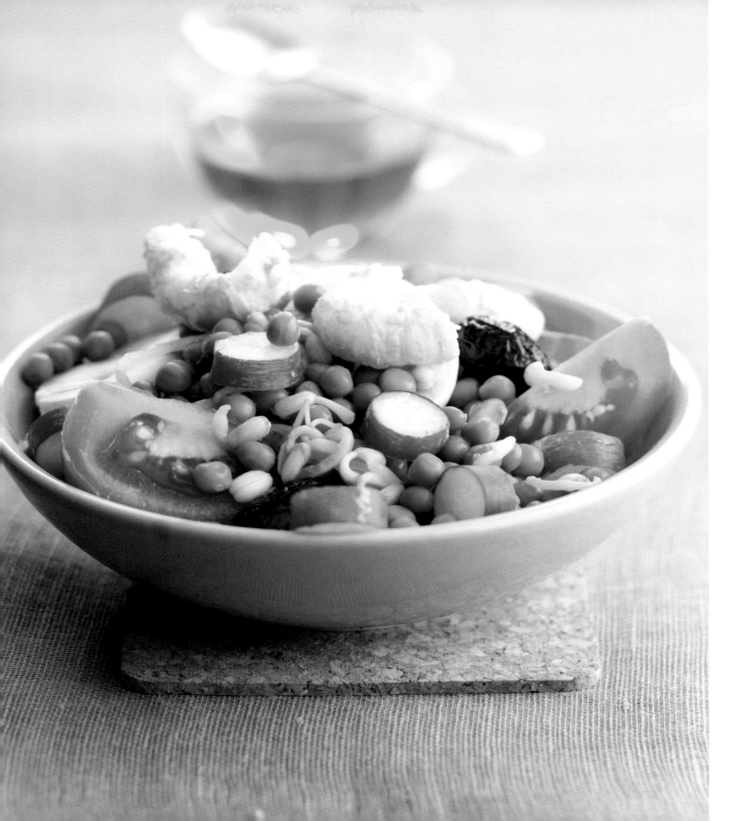

Greek Salad

Serves 4

Preparation: 15 minutes

- 1 cucumber
- 4 tomatoes
- 1 fresh white onion or 1 red anion
- 2 small green peppers
- 5oz (150 g) feta
- 24 black olives
- 1 tablespoon chopped parsley or a few leaves basil

For the vinaigrette:
- 2 tablespoons olive ail
- 1 tablespoon wine vinegar
- Salt, pepper

- Wash and quarter the tomatoes.
- Peel the cucumber and cut into medium thick slices. Do the same with the onion.
- Remove the stalk ends from the peppers, pare thinly with a potato peeler, remove the seeds and cut into pieces.
- Make a vinaigrette from the olive ail, wine vinegar, salt and pepper.
- Toss the salad ingredients in the vinaigrette and transfer to individual plates.
- Serve with slices of feta and black olives, and garnished with chopped parsley.

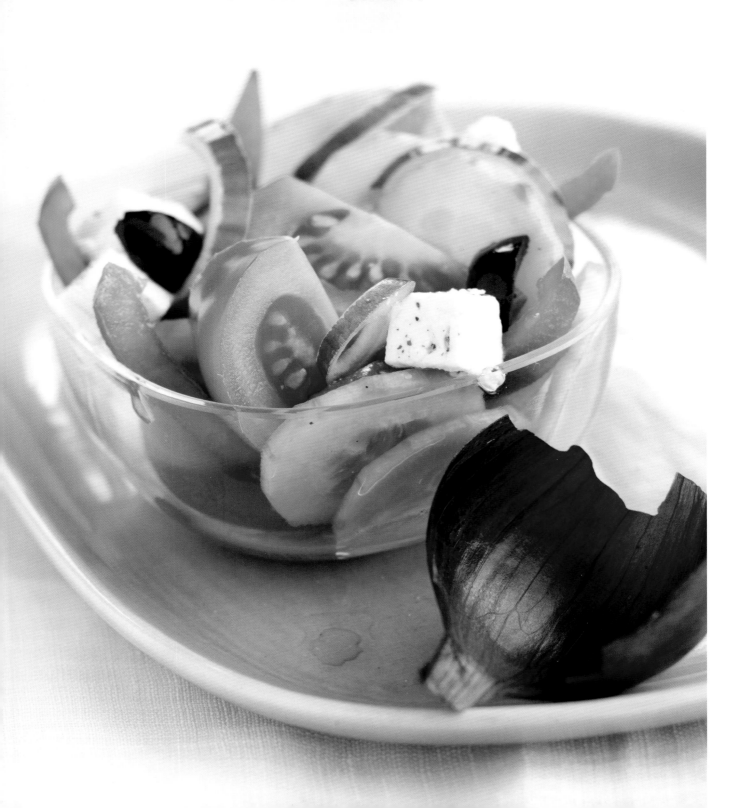

Seafood Salad

Serves 6

Preparation: 30 minutes
Cooking time: 30 minutes

- 1lb (500 g) squid
- 1/2 litre mussels
- 1/2 litre cockles
- 120 ml dry white wine
- 1 head escarole (frisée or cos)
- 3 tomatoes
- Juice of 1 lemon
- Olive oil
- Chopped fines herbs
- Salt, pepper

- Use ready-prepared squid. Clean it and cut into strips. Cook for 15 to 20 minutes in boiling water. Drain and dry.
- Wash the cockles. Heat the white wine and plunge the cockles into it, on a high heat, so that they open up. Remove from their shells and drain. (Keep the liquid.)
- Again over a high heat, open the mussels and remove from their shells. Make a sauce consisting of two thirds liquid reserved from the cockles to one third olive oil, adding the lemon juice, chopped fines herbs, salt and pepper.
- Pour this over the seafood and leave for 20 to 30 minutes.
- Shred the lettuce and transfer to the salad-bowl. Just before serving, pour the shellfish on top and garnish with tomato quarters.

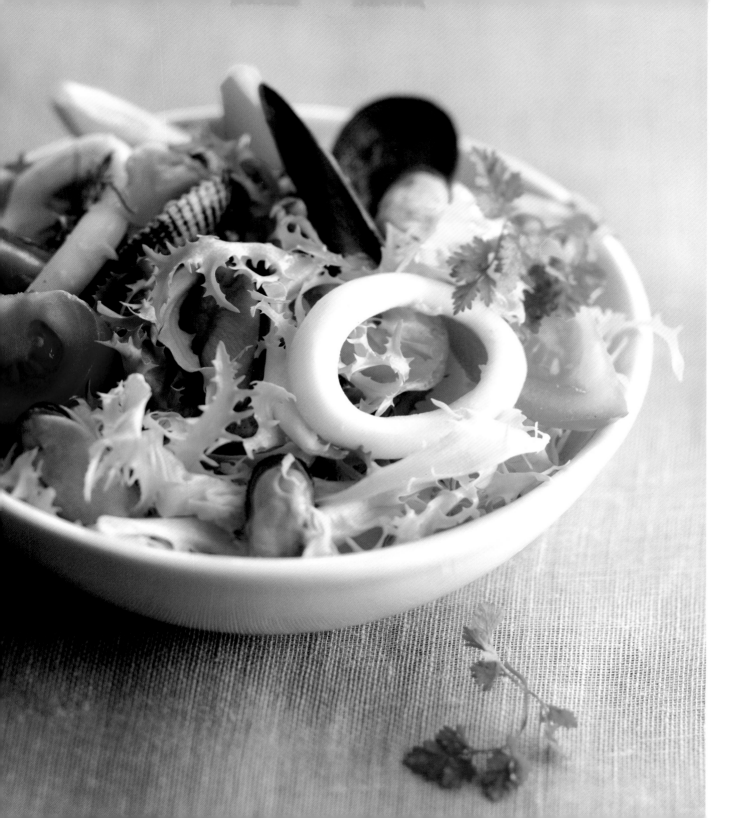

Salade niçoise
with wholegrain
Serves 6-8

Preparation: 10 minutes
Cooking time: 15 to 18 minutes
Refrigeration: 30 minutes

- 14oz (400 g) long wholegrain rice
- 1 cucumber
- 1 green and 1 red pepper
- 6 firm tomatoes
- 4oz (125 g) stoned black olives
- 2 fresh white onions
- 1 clove garlic
- 1 small tin anchovies in oil
- 2 small tins tuna in oil

For the dressing:
- 4 tablespoons olive oil
- 1 tablespoon vinegar
- 1 teaspoon mustard
- Salt, pepper

- Cook the rice in salted boiling water for 35 to 40 minutes. Rinse and drain.
- Peel the cucumber. Dice the cucumber, tomatoes, and peppers. Mix with the chopped onions, olives and the flaked tuna.
- Make a vinaigrette dressing and add to the salad
- Mix thoroughly with the rice and allow to stand in the refrigerator for 30 minutes.
- Serve chilled.

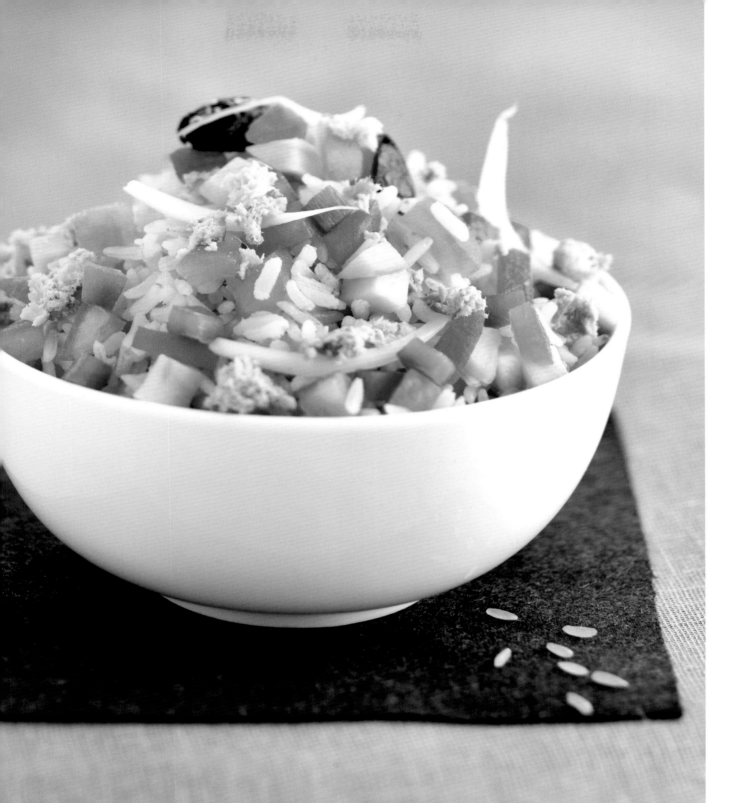

Oriental Salad

Serves 4

Preparation: 20 minutes

- 5oz (150 g) bean sprouts
- 1/2 cucumber
- 4oz (100 g) white cabbage
- 4oz (100 g) red cabbage

For the vinaigrette:
- 2 tablespoons wine vinegar
- 1 tablespoon olive oil
- 1 tablespoon bottled soy sauce
- Salt, pepper

- Wash and drain the vegetables.
- Shred the cabbage finely with a very sharp knife.
- Peel the cucumber and dice it.
- Make a vinaigrette from the oil, vinegar, soy sauce, salt and pepper.
- Mingle the vegetables together in the vinaigrette and serve chilled.

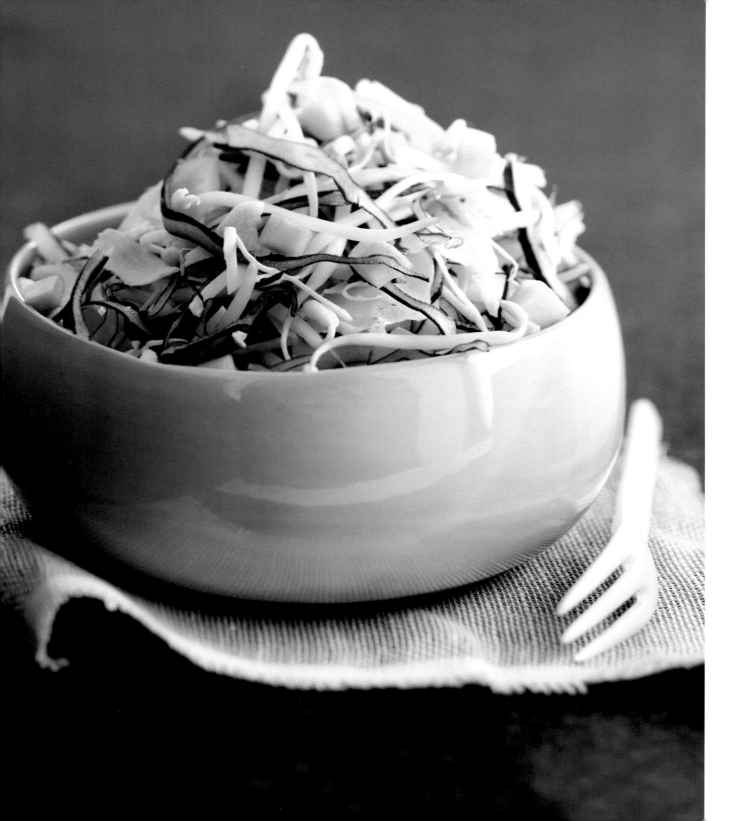

Egg, tuna and prawn salad with paprika dressing
Serves 6

Preparation: 20 minutes
Cooking time: 3 minutes

- 1 good-sized lettuce
- 6 tomatoes
- 3 hard-boiled eggs
- 7oz (200 g) tinned tuna in brine
- 7oz (200 g) frozen peeled prawns
- 14oz (400 g) fresh button mushrooms
- Juice of 1 lemon

For the vinaigrette:
- 3-4 tablespoons olive oil
- 1-2 tablespoons wine vinegar
- 1 tablespoon paprika
- Mustard
- Salt, pepper

- Trim the mushrooms as necessary wash thoroughly under cold water and drain. Slice thinly into a dish and sprinkle with lemon juice.
- If the frozen prawns are uncooked, plunge them into well salted boiling water for 3 minutes and then rinse in cold water.
- Use scissors to shred the lettuce.
- Slice the tomatoes and cut the eggs into quarters.
- Drain and flake the tuna. Put all the ingredients into a salad-bowl.
- Make a vinaigrette of olive oil, vinegar, mustard, salt and pepper and stir the paprika into it.
- Serve the vinaigrette separately.

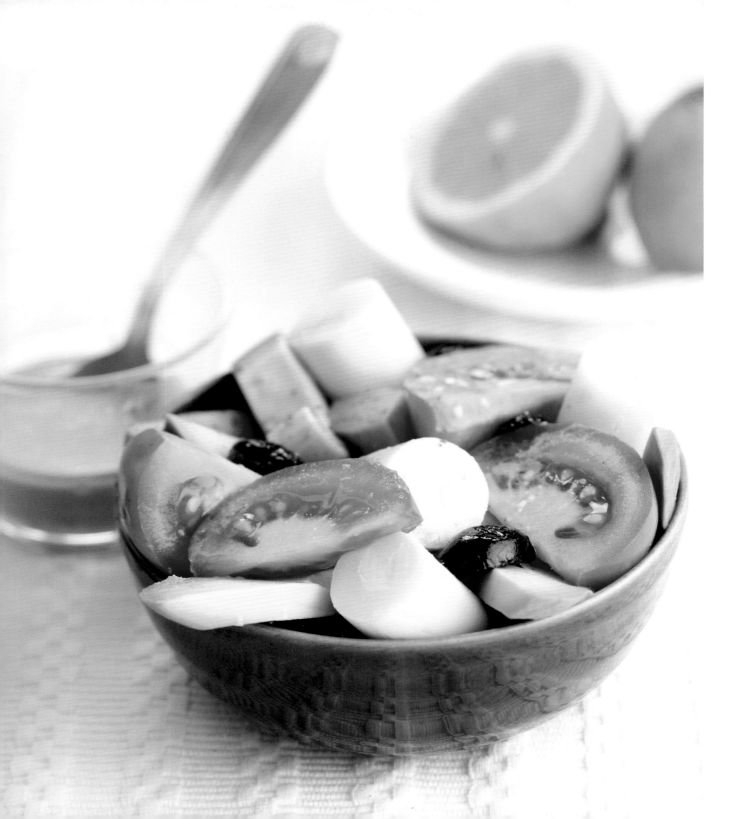

Salad of mixed summer vegetables

Serves 6

Preparation: 1 hour
Cooking time: 25 minutes
Refrigeration: 20 to 30 minutes

- 2¼ lb (1 kg) short asparagus (white or green type)
- 9oz (250 g) French beans
- Half a raw cauliflower
- 1 cucumber
- 1 bunch radishes
- 1 lettuce
- 1 medium anion
- 1 bunch chervil
- 2 sprigs tarragon
- 1 bunch watercress

For the vinaigrette :
- 4 tablespoons olive oil
- 1 tablespoon vinegar
- Salt, pepper

- Cook the beans for about 12 minutes, so they are still firm, and cut them into pieces a few centimetres long.
- Do the same with the asparagus, first peeling the stalks as necessary.
- Wash the cucumber but do not peel. Slice thinly.
- Break the cauliflower into florets and blanch for 2 minutes in boiling water.
- Make vinaigrette and add the chopped chervil, tarragon, watercress leaves, and onion.
- Wash the lettuce and shred the heart.
- Slice half the radishes.
- Mix all the ingredients together in the vinaigrette and leave in the refrigerator for 20 to 30 minutes for the flavours to mingle.
- Garnish with the rest of the radishes and serve.

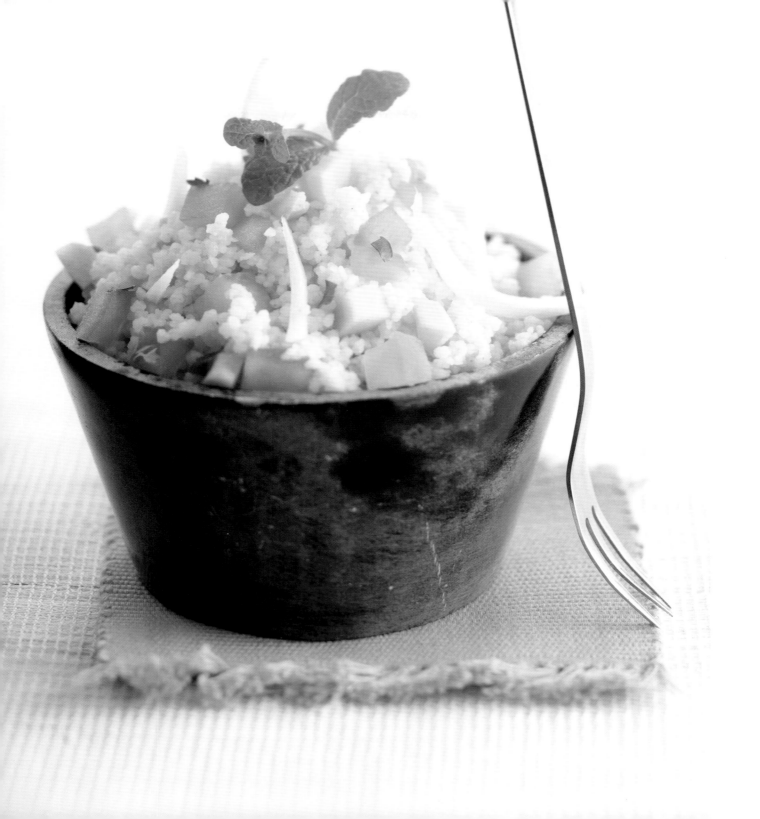

Terrine of foie gras

Serves 5

Preparation: 10 minutes
Cooking time: 55 minutes

- 2¼ lb (1 kg) fresh duck foie gras
- 4oz (100 ml) pale port
- Salt and pepper
- Nutmeg

- Place the liver in a bowl of iced water (the water should cover the liver completely) and leave in the refrigerator for 6 hours.
- Trim and season with the port, salt, pepper, and nutmeg.
- Place in a terrine dish and press well down so that it takes up the shape of the dish.
- Cover with a sheet of kitchen foil and cook in a bain-marie in a slow oven, 110 °C (220 °F, gas mark 1-2) for 35 minutes.

Suggestion :
Armagnac or sauterne may be used instead of port.

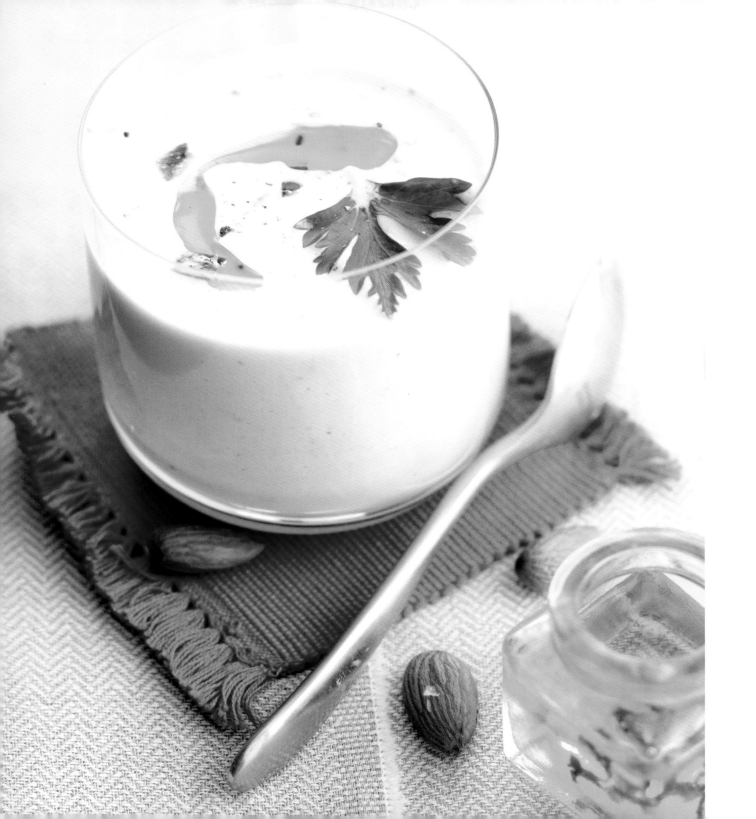

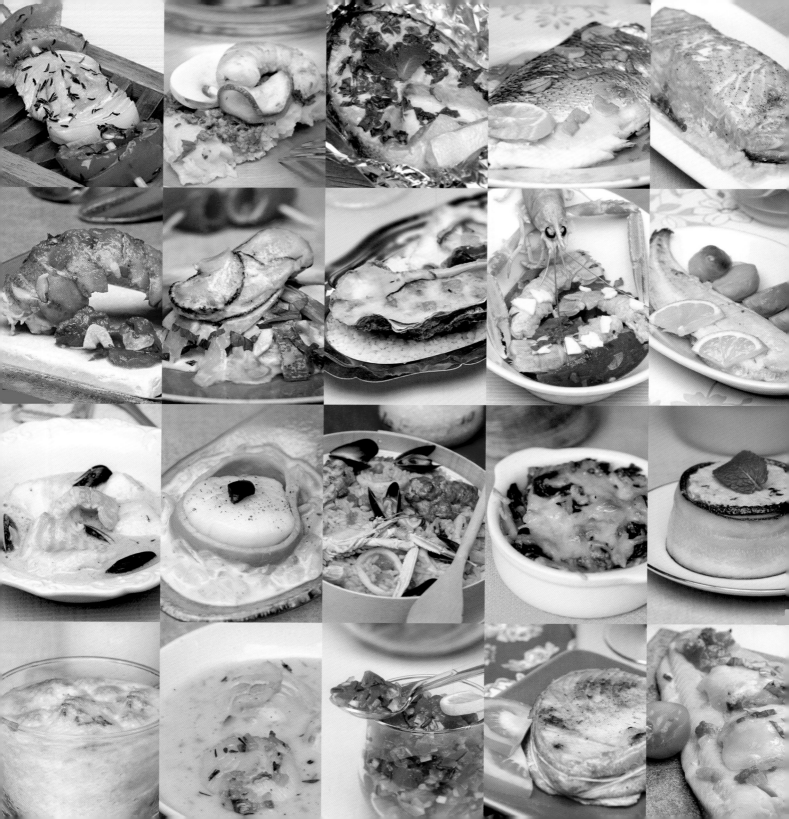

Fish recipes

Ballotins of pike
served with cabbage Serves 4

Preparation: 25 minutes
Cooking time: 20 minutes

- 18oz (500 g) pike fillets
- 9oz (250 g) fromage frais
- 4 egg whites
- 1 green cabbage
- Olive oil
- Salt, pepper

- Blend the pike fillets and combine with the fromage frais.
- Beat the egg whites until they form stiff peaks and fold in gently to give a very smooth mixture.
- Season with salt and pepper.
- Divide the mixture in four. Place each part on a piece of oiled cooking foil and roll up into a bundle. Cook for 10 minutes in the pressure cooker.
- Wash the cabbage, remove the core, and separate out the leaves. Season with salt and pepper and steam for 10 minutes.
- Spread the cabbage leaves on a serving dish and place the ballotins of fish (removed from their foil wrappings) on top.
- This dish may be served with a tomato coulis.

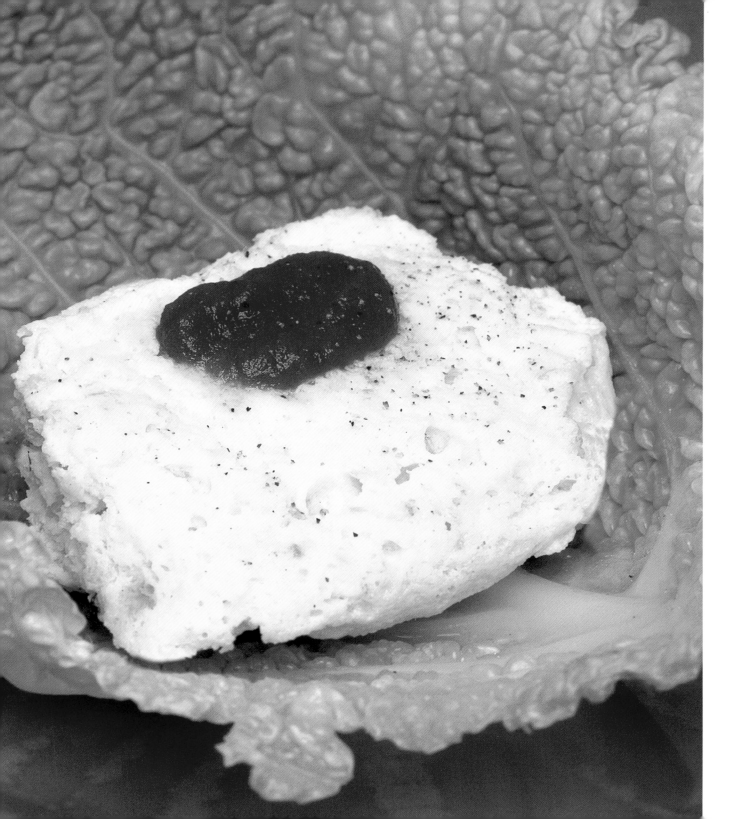

Swordfish on shewers

Serves 4

Preparation: 20 minutes
Cooking time: 15 minutes

- 2¼ lb (1 kg) of prepared swordfish
- 4 firm tomatoes
- 2 onions
- 4 green peppers
- Olive oil
- Oregano, salt, freshly ground pepper
- Herbes de Provence

- Cut the fish into 2.5cm (1in) cubes.
- Quarter the tomatoes and onions.
- Cut open the peppers, remove the stalk and seeds and cut into 2 to 3cm (1in) squares.
- Load the skewers as follows: pepper, tomato, onion, swordfish, onion, tomato…
- Arrange on an ovenware dish.
- Brush with olive oil and sprinkle with Herbes de Provence, salt, freshly ground pepper, and oregano.
- Place about 10cm (4in) under the grill and cook for about 15 minutes. Turn occasionally and baste regularly with the cooking juices.

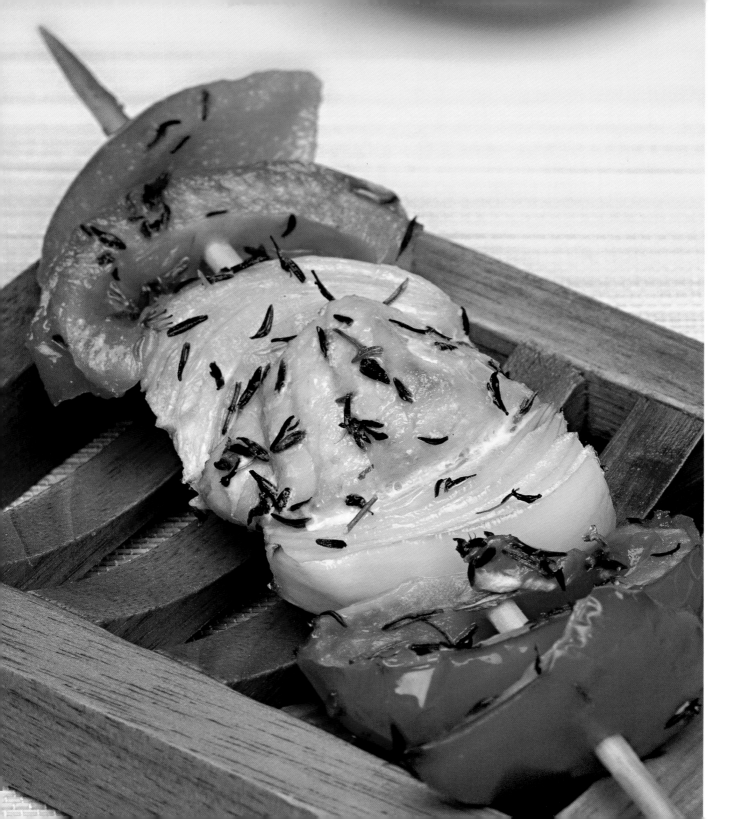

Monkfish and bacon kebabs   Serves 4

Preparation: 15 minutes
Cooking time: 15 minutes

- 2¼ lb (1 kg) monkfish
- 16 thin rashers smoked bacon
- 16 fresh bay leaves
- 2 tomatoes
- 2 lemons
- 8 small onions
- 5 tablespoons olive oil
- Salt, pepper
- Parsley

- Cut the monkfish into 16 pieces and roll each in a rasher of bacon.
- Onto each skewer thread in turn a tomato quarter, 2 pieces of monkfish, 1 bay leaf, an onion, and a lemon quarter. Repeat to complete the skewer.
- Season with salt and pepper.
- Brush the kebabs with olive oil and grill for 15 minutes.
- Serve hot, decorated with chopped parsley.

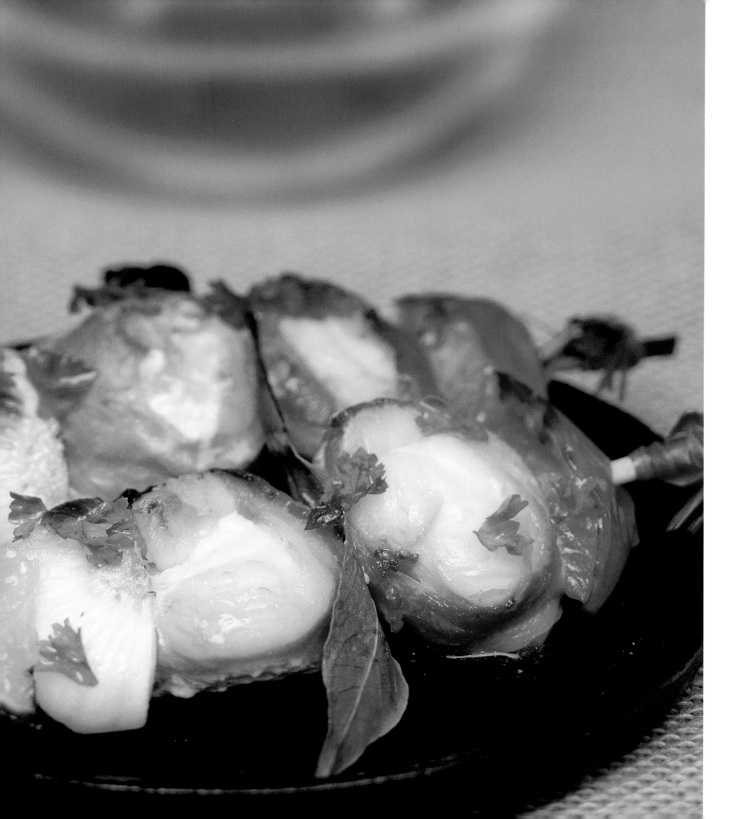

Salmon and chicken liver kebabs

Serves 6

Preparation: 30 minutes
Cooking time: 10 minutes

- 18 cubes fresh salmon
- 12 pieces chicken liver
- 2 chopped shallots
- 9oz (250 ml) low fat whipping cream or soya cream
- 13oz (37 cl) dry white wine
- Salt, pepper

- Seal the chicken livers in olive oil for 3 or 4 minutes.
- On six skewers, alternate 3 salmon cubes and 2 pieces of chicken liver.
- Place, well separated, on an oven-proof dish and season with salt and pepper.
- In a saucepan, reduce the white wine by half with the shallots on a high heat. Add the cream and simmer for 5 minutes.
- Pour this sauce over the kebabs and place the dish in the oven at 150°C (300°F, gas mark 2).
- Poach gently for 10 minutes. Remove the kebabs and keep warm.
- Reduce the cooking sauce further to obtain a thicker consistency.
- Serve the kebabs hot, accompanied by the sauce.

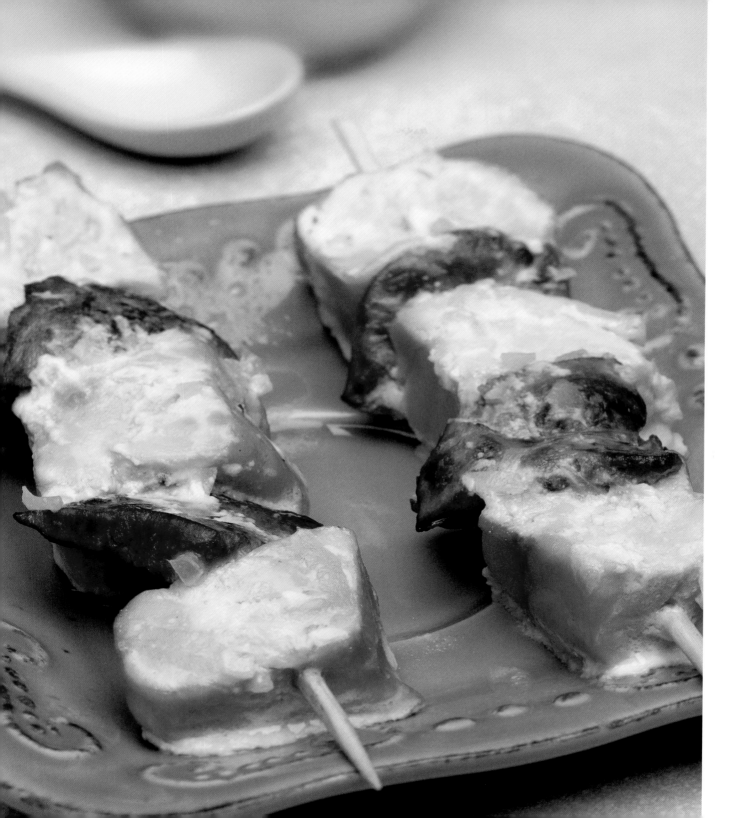

Hake with prawns and mushrooms

Serves 4

Preparation: 25 minutes
Cooking time: 35 minutes

- 2¼ lb (1 kg) hake (tail end or fillets)
- 14oz (400 g) Greenland prawns
- 9oz (250 g) fresh button mushrooms
- Soy sauce
- Chervil, coriander, parsley
- 8oz (240 ml) dry white wine
- 2¼ lb (1 kg) courgettes
- 2 onions
- Olive oil
- Coarse salt
- Salt, pepper

- Cut the hake in two to remove the central bone. Skin the fillets.
- Shell the prawns and put six to one side for decoration.
- Trim and wash the mushrooms. Blend with the prawns, parsley, chervil and half the coriander.
- Add a little soy sauce.
- Spread this mixture on the hake fillets.
- Cut the onions into rings and spread over the base of an ovenproof dish. Pour on 2 tablespoons olive oil and arrange the fish on top.
- Add the reserved prawns and the parsley. Pour the white wine over and cook in a hot oven at 200°C (400°F, gas mark 6) for 25 minutes.
- Peel the courgettes, cut into thin rings, and leave for 1 hour covered with coarse salt to draw out the water. Fry on a high heat in a little olive oil. When the courgettes are just soft, sprinkle with finely cut fresh coriander and season with salt and pepper.
- Serve the fish accompanied by the courgettes.

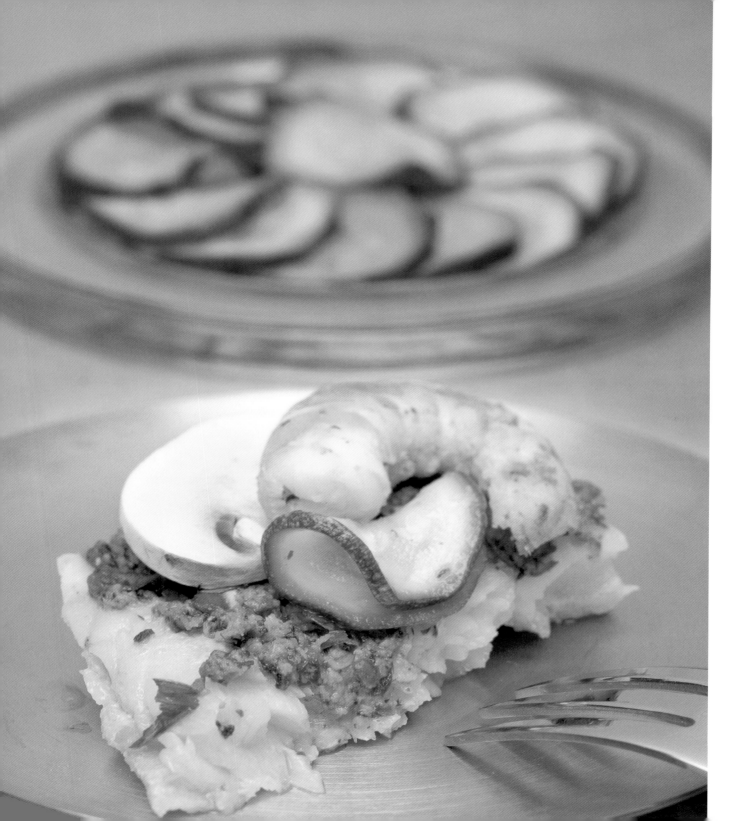

Squid provençale Serves 4 to 5

Preparation: 15 minutes
Cooking time: 45 minutes

- 2½ lb (1.25 kg) squid
- 14oz (400 g) green mild chillies
- 6 ripe tomatoes
- 5 cloves garlic
- Olive oil
- Salt, freshly ground pepper, Cayenne pepper

- Ask the fishmonger to prepare the squid, leaving just the body and the tentacles.
- Drop the tomatoes in boiling water for 1 minute before removing the skins. Halve and remove the seeds. Cut the flesh into large cubes and reduce over a very low heat in a casserole containing 2 tablespoons of olive oil. Season with salt and pepper, then reserve.
- Fry the green chillies very gently in olive oil for at least 20 minutes. Season with salt and pepper. In the last 5 minutes, add the sliced garlic and cook until pale golden, making certain it does not burn.
- Fry the tentacles and body of the squid over a gentle heat in some olive oil. Season with salt, pepper, and Cayenne pepper.
- Turn out the chillies and garlic with their cooking juices into a serving dish. Add the squid and cover with the tomato coulis. Mix well and simmer in the oven for 15 minutes in a very cool oven set at 70°C (140°F).
- Serve on warm plates.

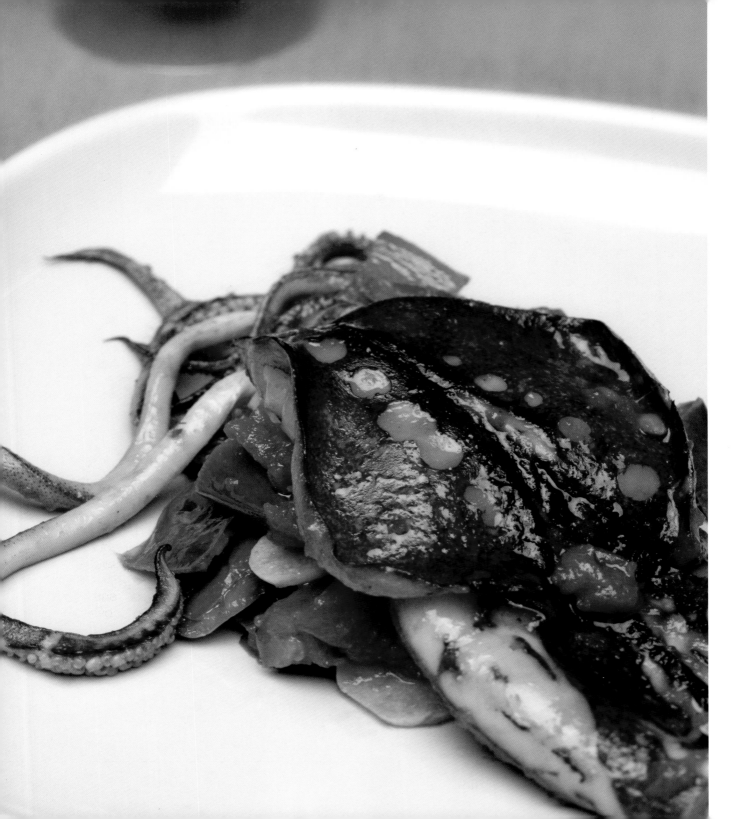

Parcels of salmon steak
with sorrel and mint

Serves 6

Preparation: 15 minutes
Cooking time: 10 minutes

- 6 salmon steaks (5oz or 150 g each)
- 18oz (500 g) tomatoes
- 11oz (300 g) sorrel
- 1 bunch mint
- 4oz (100 g) low-fat crème fraîche
- Olive oil
- Salt, pepper

- Wash the tomatoes, plunge into boiling water for 30 seconds, skin, and remove the seeds. Chop.
- Brush six pieces of cooking foil with olive oil and place a bed of tomatoes in each.
- Place the salmon steaks on top, each with some chopped sorrel, 3 fresh mint leaves and 1 teaspoon of crème fraîche, and season with salt and pepper.
- Close up the parcels and cook in a hot oven at 220°C (440°F, gas mark 7) for 12 minutes.

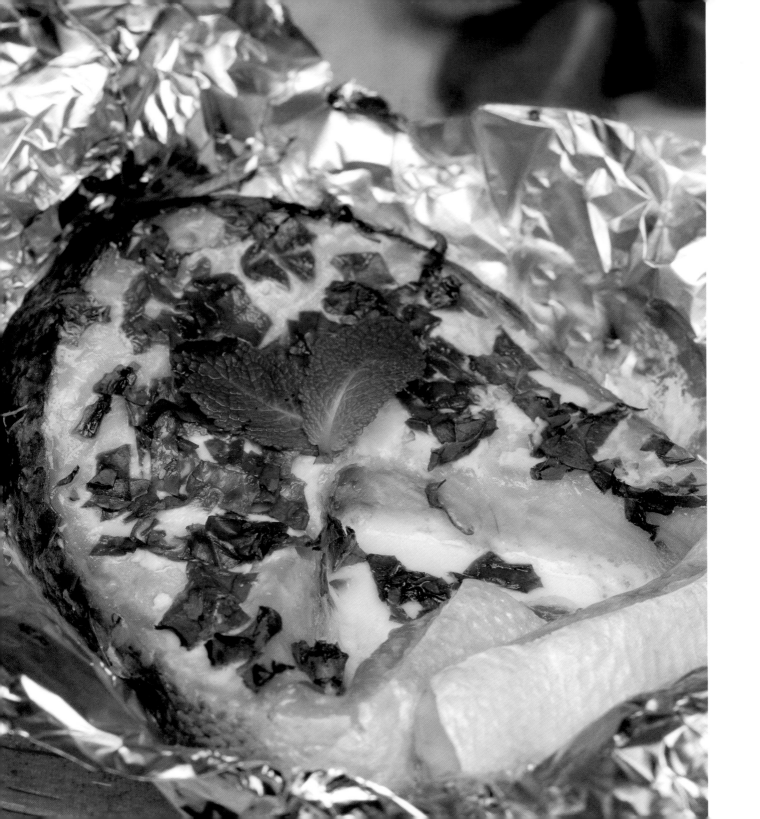

Sea bream Basque style

Serves 4

Preparation: 20 minutes
Cooking time: 25 minutes

- 2 sea bream weighing about 1¼ to 1½lb (between 600 and 700 g) each
- 5 cloves garlic – sliced thinly
- ½ glass sherry vinegar
- 2 lemons
- Olive oil
- 1 bunch parsley
- Salt, freshly ground pepper, Cayenne pepper

- Ask the fishmonger to scale and clean the bream.
- Stuff with parsley and 2 or 3 lemon slices. Season with salt, pepper, and Cayenne pepper.
- Arrange in an ovenware dish, brush with olive oil and place in the oven at 190°C (380°F, gas mark 5).
- Cook for 20 minutes – turning after 10 minutes, to cook the other side.
- Fillet the sea bream. Arrange on warm plates. Squeeze lemon juice over the top and reserve in a warm place.
- Immediately put the sliced garlic in a pan with 3 tablespoons olive oil. Cook until barely golden. Season with salt, pepper, and Cayenne pepper. At the last moment, add the sherry vinegar.
- After 30 seconds, pour the boiling sauce over the fish and serve at once.

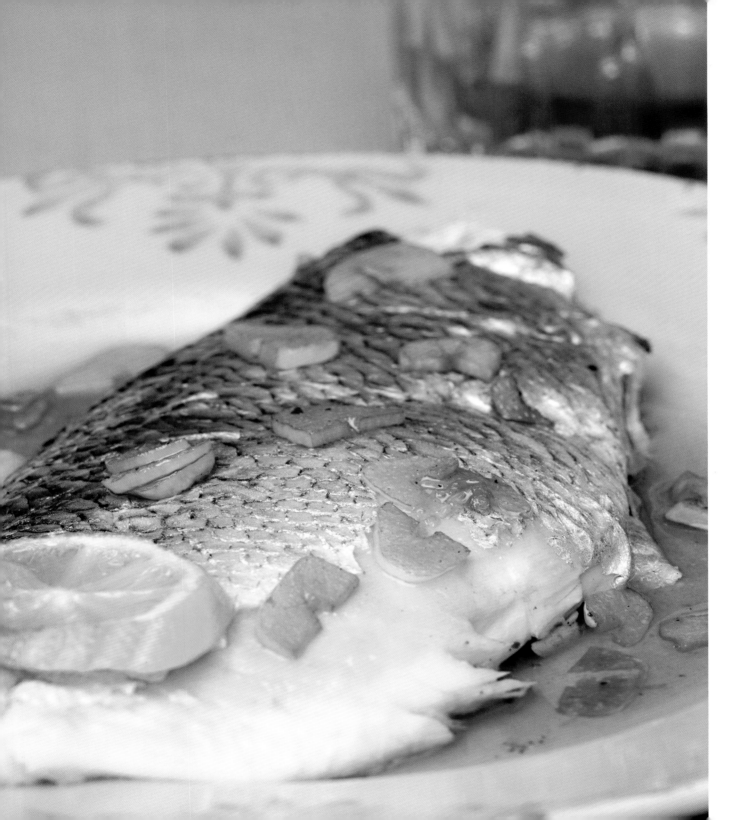

Sea bass fillets
with shallot sauce

Serves 4

Preparation: 20 minutes
Cooking time: 55 minutes

- 2¼ lb (1 kg) sea bass fillets
- 4 shallots
- 2 tablespoons olive oil
- 7fl oz (20 cl) double cream

For the fish stock:
- Head and bones
- 1 onion
- 1 stick of celery
- 2 sprigs parsley
- 1 bouquet garni
- ½ glass dry white wine
- ½ glass red wine vinegar
- Salt, pepper

- Ask the fishmonger to prepare the fillets and reserve the head and bones for making the fish stock.
- To prepare the fish stock, chop up the onion, celery and parsley.
- Tip into 1.5 litres of water together with the bouquet garni, and boil for 30 minutes. Add the white wine and the vinegar. Allow to cool and pass through a conical strainer.
- Add the fish head and bones to the stock. Bring to the boil and continue to reduce over a low heat, until all that remains is a glassful. Season with salt and pepper.
- Liquidize the shallots and mix with the olive oil.
- In an ovenware dish that has been lightly oiled, place the fillets with the skin side downwards. Season with salt and pepper. Spread the shallot and oil mixture on the fillets.
- Place in the oven about 10cm (4ln) below the grill, and cook for 6 to 7 minutes.
- Mix the glass of fish stock with the double cream. Check seasoning.
Cook gently for a further 1 minute.
- Coat the fillets with the sauce and serve.

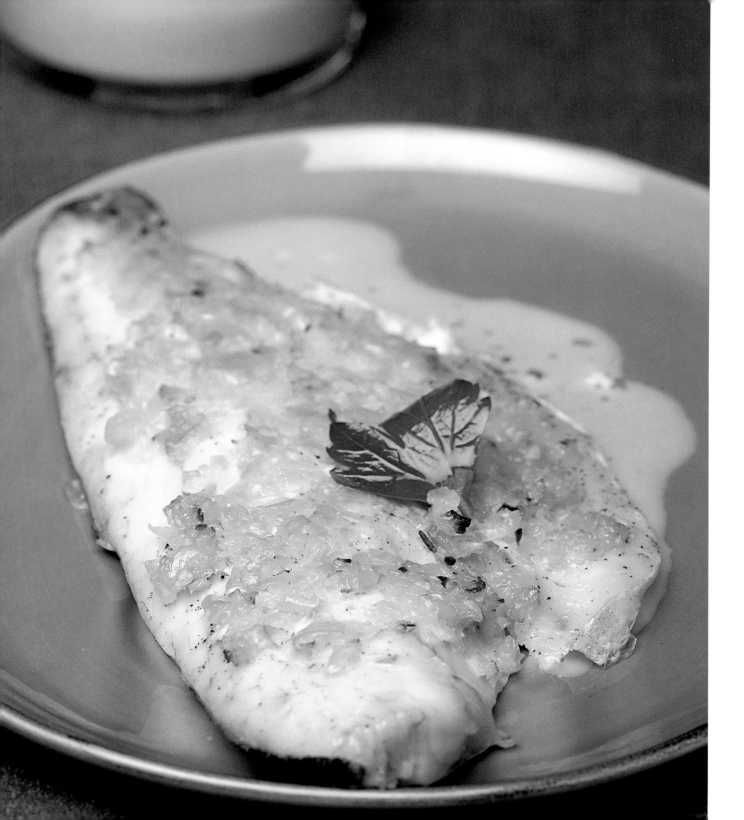

Parcels of salmon fillet with puree of green peppers Serves 4

Preparation: 15 minutes
Cooking time: 45 minutes

- 4 salmon fillets (5oz or 150 g each)
- 2 new onions
- 2 tablespoons low-fat crème fraîche
- 4 to 5 green peppers
- 1 lemon
- 5 tablespoons dry white wine
- Salt, pepper

- Wrap the peppers in cooking foil and bake in a hot oven at 250°C (500°F, gas mark 9) for 45 minutes.
- Meanwhile, cook the sliced onions in the white wine until it has evaporated.
- Season the fish with salt and pepper and squeeze a few drops of lemon over it.
- Wrap immediately in envelopes of cooking foil. Bake in a hot oven at 250°C (500°F, gas mark 9) for 15 minutes.
- Peel the peppers, cut them in half, and blend with the onions and crème fraîche.
- Adjust the seasoning and serve the salmon surrounded by the puree of peppers.

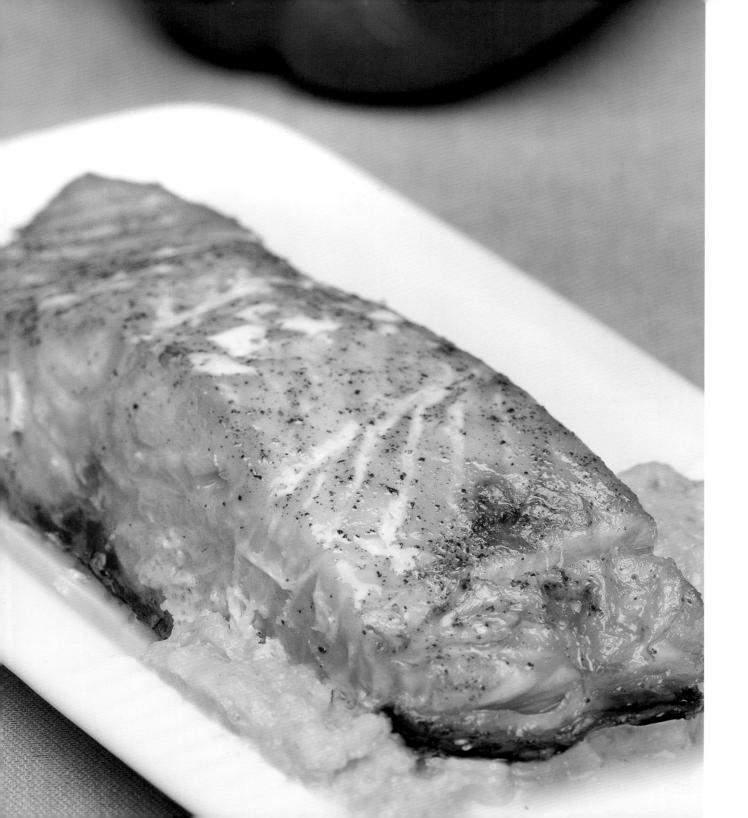

Grilled salmon fillets with Tamari

Serves 4

Preparation: 10 minutes
Cooking time: 10 minutes

- 1¾ lb (800 g) salmon fillets
- 1 lemon
- Olive oil
- Tamari (thick soy sauce)
- Fine sea salt
- Pepper, Herbes de Provence
- 1 tablespoon chopped parsley

- Cut the fillets into 4 equal pieces. Brush with olive oil. Season with salt and pepper.
- Pre-heat the oven grill.
- Place the fillet pieces in an ovenware dish with the skin facing uppermost. Sprinkle lightly with Herbes de Provence.
- Cook under the grill for 10 minutes.
- Meanwhile, prepare the sauce: 1/3 lemon juice, 1/3 olive oil, 1/3 tamari, a pinch of sea salt and a pinch of pepper.
- Arrange the salmon on the plates, with the skin side down. Sprinkle with chopped parsley. Stir the sauce well, pour over the top and serve.

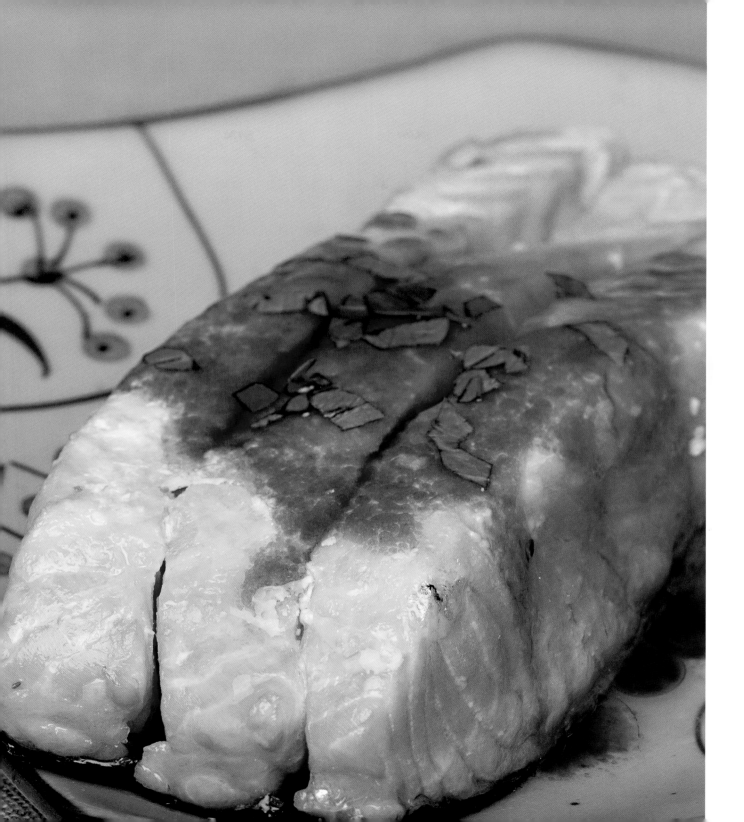

Fillets of sole
with soya cream Serves 4

Preparation: 20 minutes
Cooking time: 20 minutes

- 4 large fillets of sole
- Juice of 1 lemon
- 5oz (150 g) button mushrooms, washed, and sliced
- 7fl oz (20 cl) soya cream
- 4oz (100 g) peeled prawns
- 1 egg yolk
- Olive oil
- Salt, freshly ground pepper
- 1 tablespoon fresh parsley

- Wash the fillets under the tap and pat dry with absorbent kitchen paper.
- Heat 2 tablespoons of olive oil in a non-stick frying pan, and gently fry the fish. Pour lemon juice over the top. Season with salt and pepper. Continue cooking over a low heat for 2 minutes. Set aside and keep warm.
- Fry the mushrooms over a gentle heat in 2 tablespoons of olive oil.
- Discard the cooking juices and the water from the mushrooms. Add the soya cream, mixed beforehand in a bowl with the egg yolk. Season with salt and pepper. Add the prawns.
- Continue cooking over a low heat for a few minutes, stirring continuously.
- Arrange the fish on warmed plates and coat with the sauce. Sprinkle with chopped parsley and serve.

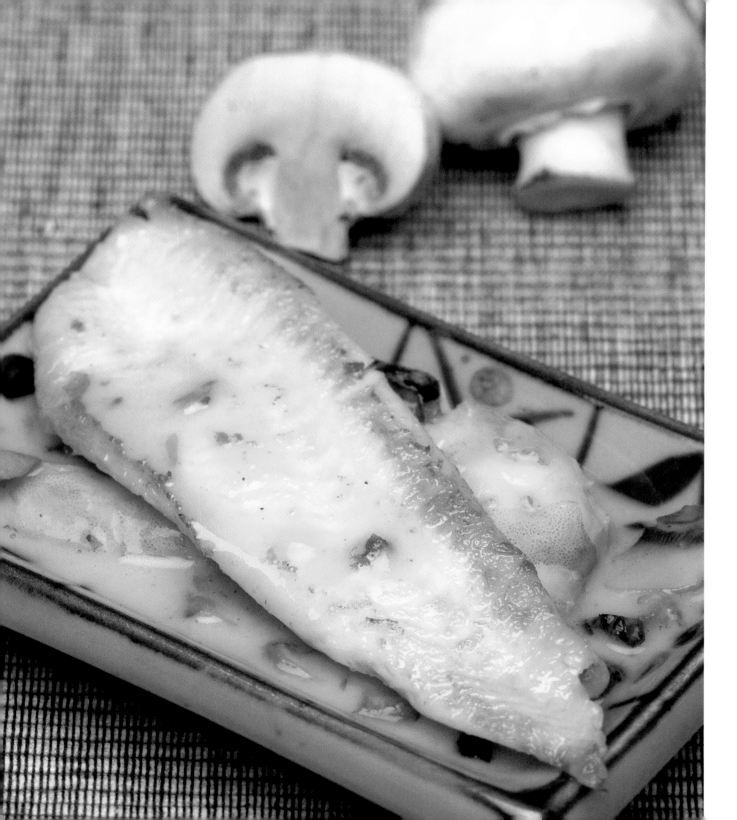

Fillets of sole with an aubergine puree

Serves 4

Preparation: 20 minutes
Cooking time: 30 minutes

- 4 sole fillets (5 oz or 150 g each)
- 1 to 2 ladles of court-bouillon
- 2¼ lb (1 kg) aubergines
- 1 lemon
- 4oz (100 ml) olive oil
- 4 basil leaves
- Salt, pepper

- Grill the aubergines for 30 minutes, turning during this time, so that all the skin is well done (almost burnt).
- Remove the skin and seeds and blend the flesh with the olive oil, lemon juice, basil, salt, and pepper.
- Arrange the sole fillets in an ovenproof dish. Pour the court-bouillon over and cook in a hot oven at 200°C (400°F, gas mark 6) for 5 to 7 minutes.
- Arrange the sole fillets on a warmed serving dish with the aubergine purée around them.

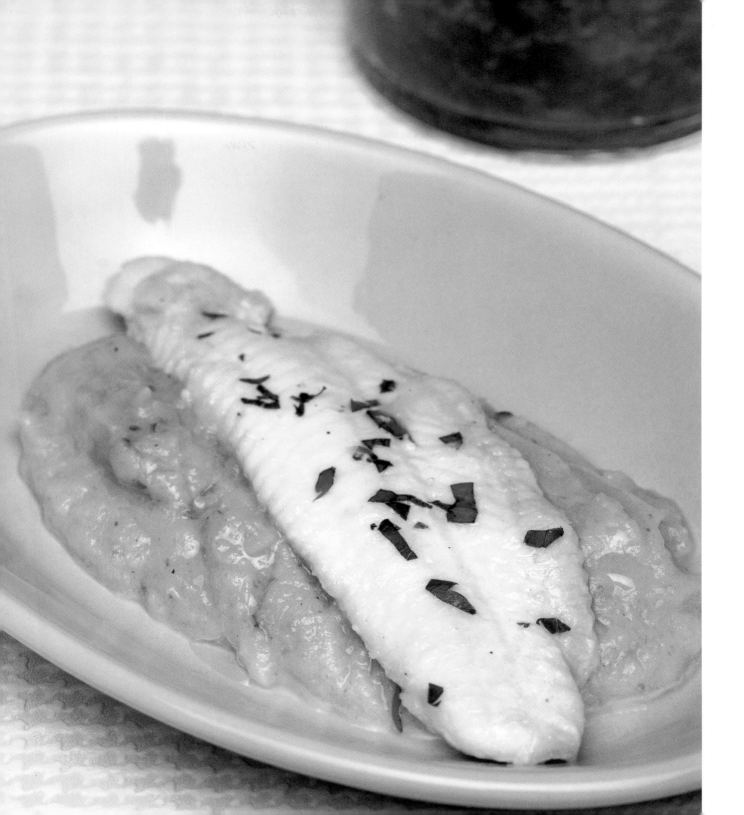

Fillets of sole with salmon

Serves 4

Preparation: 15 minutes
Cooking time: 20 minutes

- 4 good sized soles
- 10oz (300 g) fillet of salmon
- 5 shallots – sliced
- 3 tablespoons low fat crème fraîche or soya cream
- 5fl oz (15 cl) dry white wine
- Juice of ½ lemon
- 1 tablespoon freshly chopped parsley
- Salt, pepper

- Ask the fishmonger to fillet the sole and then to slice the salmon fillets thinly as for smoked salmon.
- Take a fillet of sole and cover with a fillet of salmon and roll the two together. Secure by spiking with a wooden toothpick.
- In a pan, brown the shallots a few minutes in olive oil. Then add the white wine. Season with salt and pepper and cook for 1 minute.
- Put the fish rolls in an ovenware dish. Season with salt and pepper. Pour the wine mixture over the top.
- Place in a fairly hot oven at 190°C (380°F, gas mark 5) for 12 to 15 minutes.
- Take out of the oven and arrange the fish on a serving dish. Reserve in warm place.
- Quickly add the crème fraîche and the lemon juice to the cooking juices in the ovenware dish and blend with a fork.
- Coat the fish rolls with the sauce and decorate with parsley before serving.

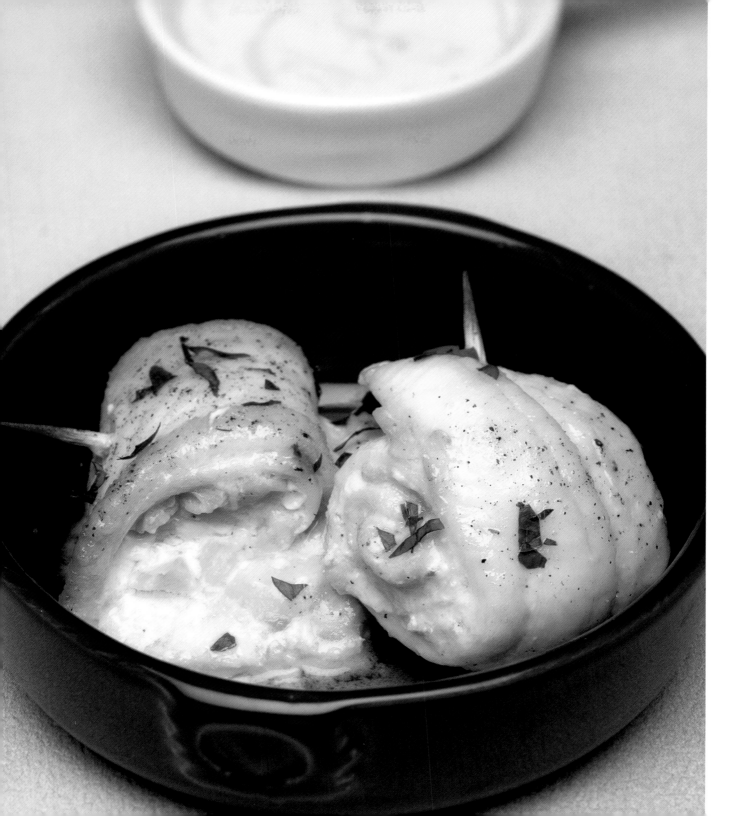

Goose foie gras
with scallops   Serves 6

Preparation: 1 hour
Cooking time: 30 minutes

- 1 fresh foie gras (28oz or 800 g)
- 8 good-sized scallops
- 1/2 glass port
- Salt, sweet paprika

- Clean the scallops and open them by placing over a high heat for a few seconds. Separate the white parts from the corals (roes) and slice the whites thinly. Season with salt and sweet paprika.
- Blend the corals to a purée with the port and some sweet paprika.
- Place the foie gras in iced water for 6 hours. Trim and season with salt and pepper.
- Place some of the scallop in the bottom of a terrine dish and lay the foie gras on top. Press down well so that it takes up the shape of the dish. Pour the coral purée over and cover with the remaining scallop slices.
- Cover with a sheet of kitchen foil and cook in a bain-marie in a slow oven at 120°C (240°F, gas mark ¼) for 35 minutes.
- Serve lukewarm.

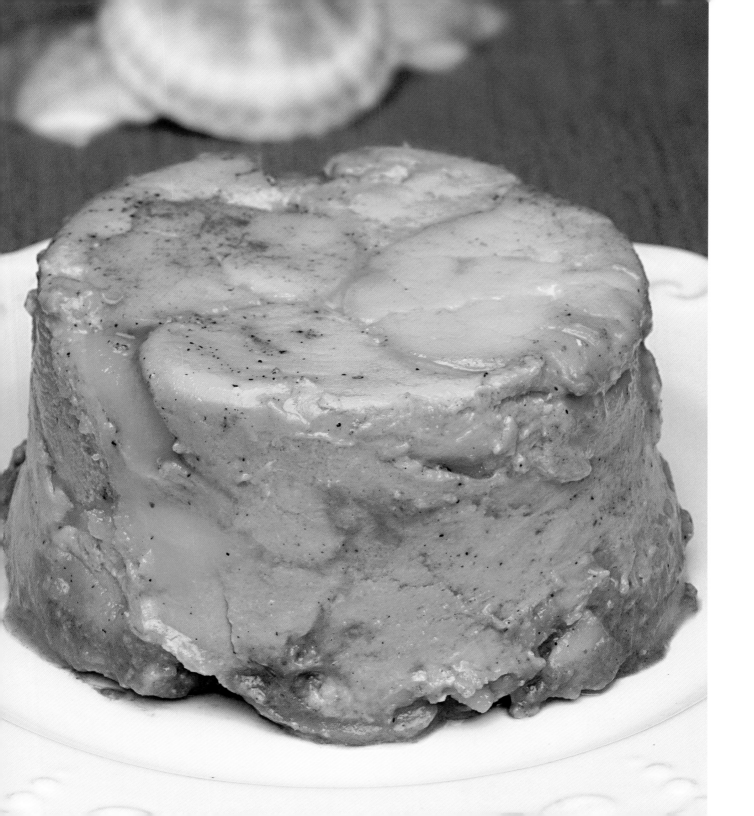

Sauteed prawns
with ratatouille   Serves 4

Preparation: 20 minutes
Cooking time: 20 minutes

- 24 large prawns
- 1 aubergine
- 2 courgettes
- 3 tomatoes
- 1/2 red pepper
- 1/2 green pepper

- 1/2 yellow pepper
- 2 cloves garlic
- 3 sprigs parsley
- Coriander seeds
- 3 tablespoons olive oil
- 1 tablespoon coarse salt

- Plunge the tomatoes into boiling water for 30 seconds, skin and remove the seeds. Seed the peppers and dice finely, but do not peel. Dice the aubergines and courgettes finely.
- Using a non-stick pan, cover and sweat each type of vegetable separately for 10 minutes on a low heat.
- Chop the garlic clove and the parsley.
- Put all the vegetables together in a skillet and fry on a high heat for 1 to 2 minutes in 2 tablespoons of olive oil.
- Shell the raw prawns and remove the heads and toils.
- Heat 2 tablespoons of olive oil with the salt and fry on a high heat for 2 minutes. Turn the prawns over and sprinkle with garlic and chopped parsley. Add the coriander and leave for one more minute.
- Serve 5 or 6 prawns per plate with a little ratatouille.

Suggestion:
Frozen prawns are perfectly satisfactory for this recipe.

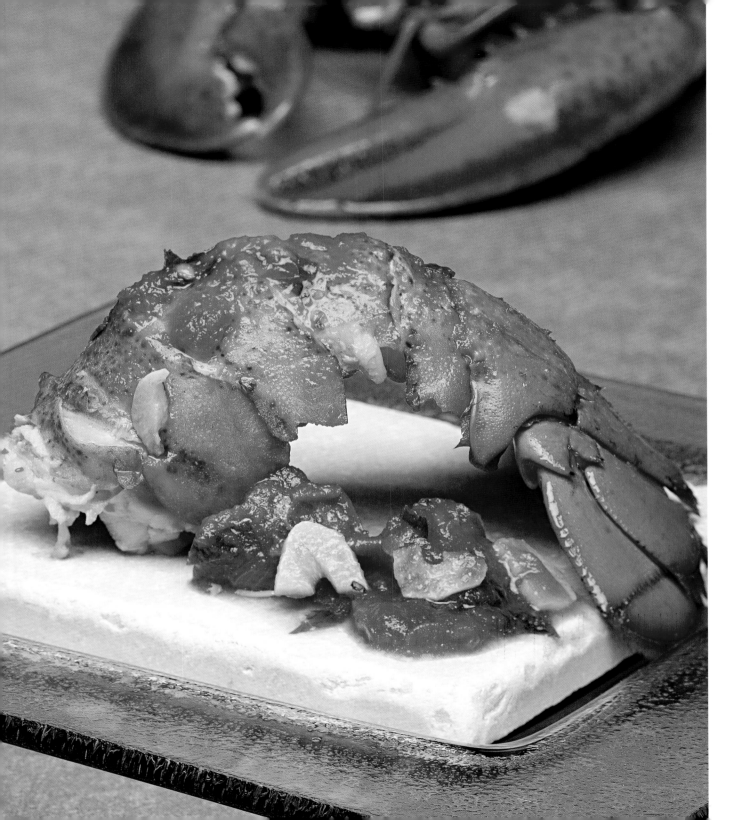

Oysters served hot with raw ham

Serves 4

Preparation: 10 minutes
Cooking time: 18 minutes

- 4 dozen good-sized oysters
- 2 good-sized slices raw ham
- 2 shallots, finely chopped
- 7oz (200 g) fresh mushrooms, sliced
- 1 tablespoon lemon juice
- 2 pinches celery salt
- 4oz (100 ml) law-fat crème fraîche
- 2 tablespoons chopped parsley
- Salt, pepper

- Open the oysters and remove from the shells. Filter the liquid.
- Cut the ham into strips and fry on a high heat. Add the liquid from the oysters, together with the shallots, the sliced mushrooms, lemon juice, salt, pepper and celery salt. Cover and simmer for 5 minutes. Uncover and simmer for a further 5 minutes to reduce the cooking liquid.
- Add the oysters and bring to the boil. Finally stir in the cream, sprinkle with parsley and leave over the heat for a further minute, stirring all the time.
- Serve at once on warmed plates.

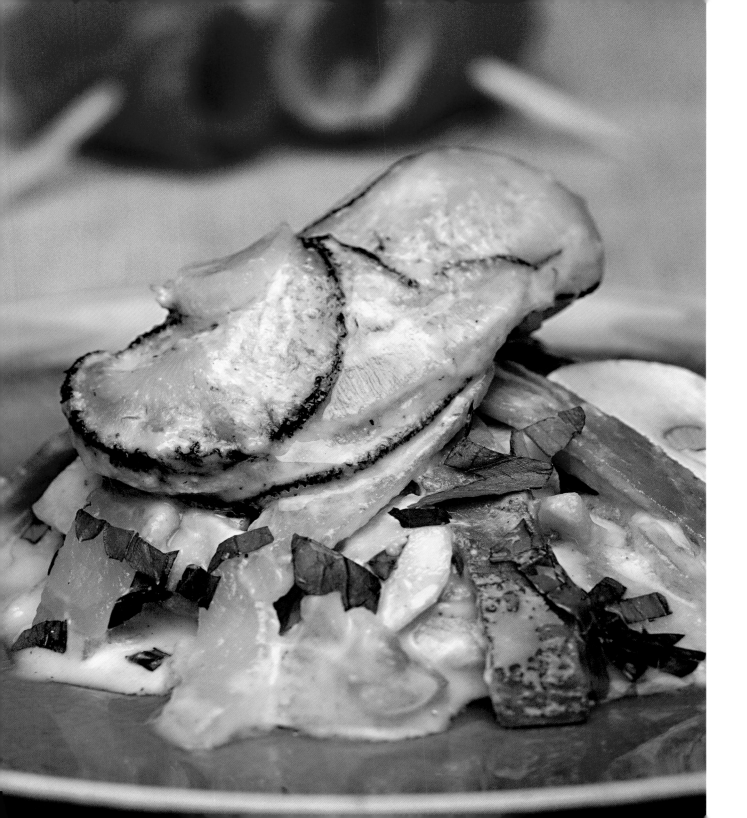

Oysters in a sabayon

Serves 4

Preparation: 20 minutes
Cooking time: 5 minutes

- 24 oysters (preferably from Marennes or Oléron)
- 6 egg yolks
- 14oz (400 g) tomatoes
- 1 lemon
- 1 tablespoon finely chopped chives
- 3 tablespoons low-fat whipping cream
- Coarse salt, pepper

- Open the oysters and detach from their shells, but leave in the shells. Collect 150 ml (5oz) of the liquid and filter it.
- Plunge the tomatoes into boiling water for 30 seconds, skin and remove the seeds. Dice the flesh and leave to drain in a colander.
- In a bain-marie, gently heat the egg yolks and the liquid from the oysters, whisking with an electric hand-whisk. Turn the heat up as the mixture begins to froth up.
- Season the whipped mixture with the pepper and chives. Add the whipped cream and a few drops of lemon juice.
- Preheat the grill.
- Divide the diced tomatoes among the oysters and spoon the sabayon mixture on top.
- Place the sea salt in an ovenproof dish to make a bed on which the oysters can be placed. Grill for 1 minute.
- Serve immediately.

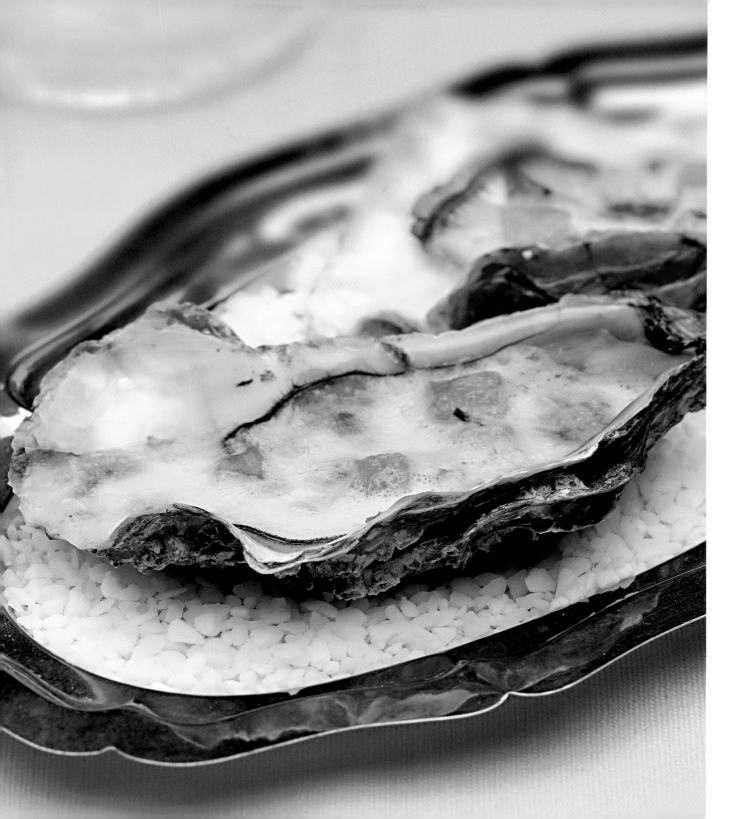

Poached oysters
on a bed of leeks   Serves 4

Preparation: 20 minutes
Cooking time: 25 minutes

- 2 dozen medium oysters
- 3 leek whites
- 3 tablespoons low fat crème fraîche or soya cream
- 3 shallots – sliced
- 1 glass dry white wine
- Olive oil
- Salt, freshly ground pepper

- In a casserole, brown the shallots with 1 tablespoon of olive oil. Add the white wine.
- Season with salt and pepper. Reduce by a third and reserve.
- Clean the leeks. Cut each leek into 2 or 3 sections and then slice down their length into juliennes. Fry over a low heat in olive oil. Cover and sweat. Reserve and keep warm
- Open the oysters (use a steel glove and special knife if possible, to avoid the risk of injury).
- Detach them from their shells and conserve half the liquid, adding it to the wine mixture.
- Place the casserole over a medium heat and poach the oysters for 2 minutes. Remove them with a slotted spoon, reserve and keep warm.
- Reduce the cooking juices to a quarter. Turn down the heat and add the crème fraîche. Season with pepper.
- Lay a bed of leeks on each individual plate and arrange the oysters on top, coating with the sauce.
- Serve immediately.

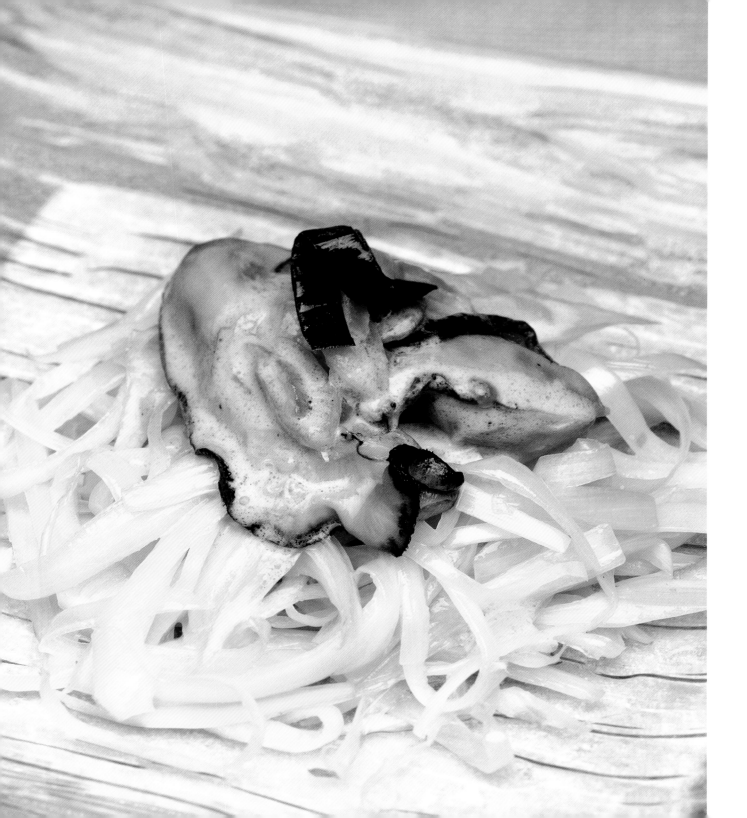

Greek-style scampi

Serves 6 to 8

Preparation: 15 minutes
Cooking time: 40 minutes

- 36 to 48 scampi (Dublin Bay prawns, langoustines)
- 2 large tins skinned tomatoes
- 4oz (120 g) feta cheese
- 2 chopped onions
- 1 large bunch parsley
- 7oz (200 ml) dry white wine
- 2 tablespoons olive oil
- 1 teaspoon oregano
- Salt, pepper

- Shell the scampi, retaining only the tail. Rinse under running water and dry on kitchen paper.
- Fry the chopped onions on a low heat in the olive oil. Add the tinned tomatoes, drained, the white wine, half the chopped parsley, the oregano and the salt and pepper. Simmer, uncovered, until the liquid has evaporated.
- Place the scampi in a pan with the rest of the olive oil. When golden brown, drain.
Add to the tomatoes little by little and sprinkle with thinly sliced feta.
- Cook for 5 minutes, stirring very gently.
- Serve decorated with chopped parsley.

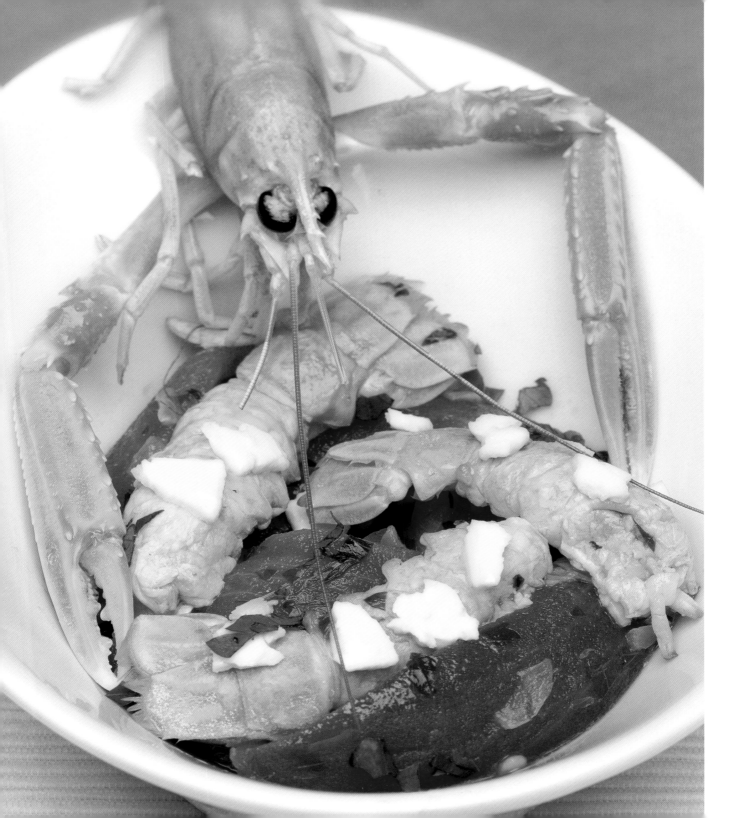

Lemon sole Cretan style

Serves 4

Preparation: 10 minutes
Cooking time: 10 minutes

- 6 lemon sole fillets
- 3 onions – sliced
- 3 lemons
- 4 bay leaves
- 2 sprigs thyme
- 1 glass olive oil
- Salt, freshly ground pepper

- Prepare a marinade with the olive oil, sliced onions, lemon juice, thyme, bay leaf, salt and pepper.
- Marinade the fish fillets for 20 minutes.
- Then pour the marinade in a frying pan over a medium heat. When the marinade is hot, add the fillets and poach for 5 minutes each side.
- Serve with a dressing of olive oil and lemon juice according to taste.

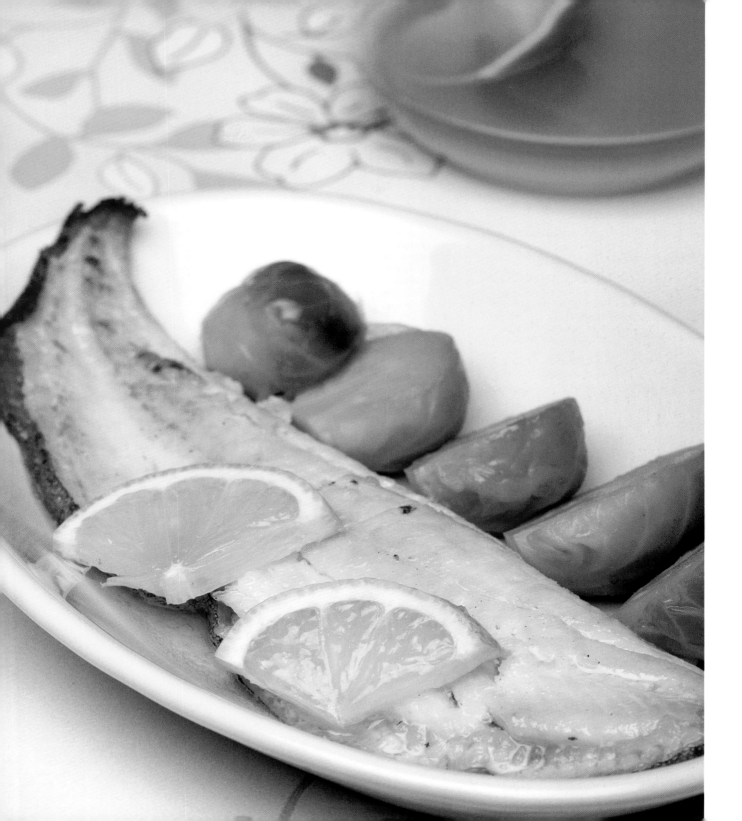

Poached mackerel with leeks

Serves 4

Preparation: 30 minutes
Cooking time: 10 minutes

- 4 mackerels (11 oz or 300 g each)
- 18oz (1/2 litre) white wine
- 4 leeks (white parts only)
- 4oz (100 g) law-fat crème fraîche
- 1 tablespoon chopped parsley
- Olive ail
- Salt, pepper

- Clean the mackerel Heat the white wine and poach the mackerel in it for 5 minutes.
- Wash the leeks and slice thinly.
- Fry in 2 tablespoons olive oil, then add a little white wine, cover and simmer for 5 minutes.
- Add the crème fraîche, salt, and pepper just before removing from the heat.
- Serve the fish decorated with chopped parsley and garnished with leeks.

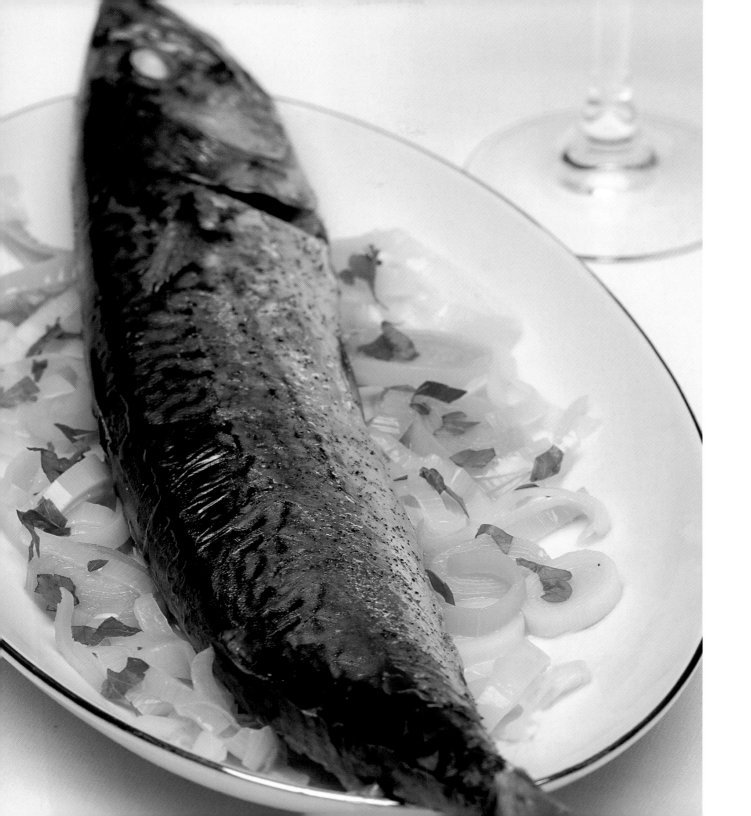

Curried mussel stew

Serves 6

Preparation: 20 minutes
Cooking time: 20 minutes

- 2 litres mussels
- 2oz (50 ml) olive oil
- 4oz (100 ml) milk
- 4oz (100 g) tinned button mushrooms
- 3 shallots
- 4 egg yolks
- 1 teaspoon curry powder
- 1 lemon
- 1 bouquet garni
- Salt, pepper
- 9oz (250 ml) low-fat crème fraîche
- 4oz (120 ml) dry white wine

- Heat the white wine, with the bouquet garni, and add the mussels, on a high heat, so that they open. Remove the upper part of the shells. Place the mussels on a dish and leave in a warm place. Strain the cooking fluid and put on one side.
- Slice the shallots and fry in olive oil, without allowing them to brown.
- Put the mushrooms through the food processor to purée them and add to the shallots.
- Stir, and then add the warmed milk, the cooking fluid, and the egg yolks. Season with salt, pepper, the curry powder, and the lemon juice.
- Cook for 10 minutes, stirring continuously. Then stir in the crème fraîche. Pour the mixture over the mussels.
- Place in a hot oven for 10 to 20 minutes and serve at once.

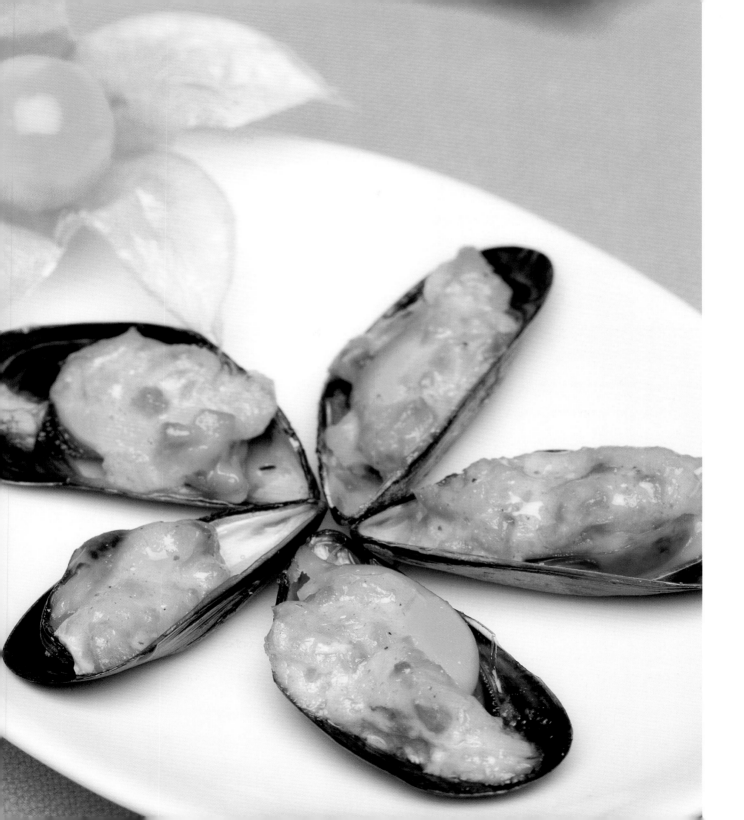

Salmon fillets in white fish mousse with mayonnaise

Serves 8 to 10

Preparation: 30 minutes
Cooking time: 1 hour 30 minutes

- 2¼ lb (1 kg) fresh salmon fillets
- 2¼ lb (1 kg) coley (or cod) fillets
- 4 egg whites
- 4oz (100 g) law-fat crème fraîche
- 7oz (200 g) mayonnaise
- 1 handful sorrel
- Salt, pepper

For the mayonnaise:
- 1 egg yolk
- 1 teaspoon mustard
- 7oz (200 ml) oil (sunflower and olive)
- A little vinegar
- Salt, pepper

- Clean the coley (or cod) fillets, put them through the blender with the sorrel and season with salt and pepper.
- Then add the crème fraîche.
- Beat the egg whites until they form stiff peaks and fold them gently into the mixture.
- Line a loaf tin with aluminium foil. Place a layer of the coley (or cod) mixture in the bottom.
- On top place some of the salmon fillets, cut as necessary, and repeat the operation until the mould has been filled.
- Cook in bain-marie in a gentle oven at 150° C (300°F, gas mark 2) for 1 hour.
- Make a classic mayonnaise with sunflower oil, adding a tablespoon of olive oil.
- Turn out the mousse and serve cold with the mayonnaise.

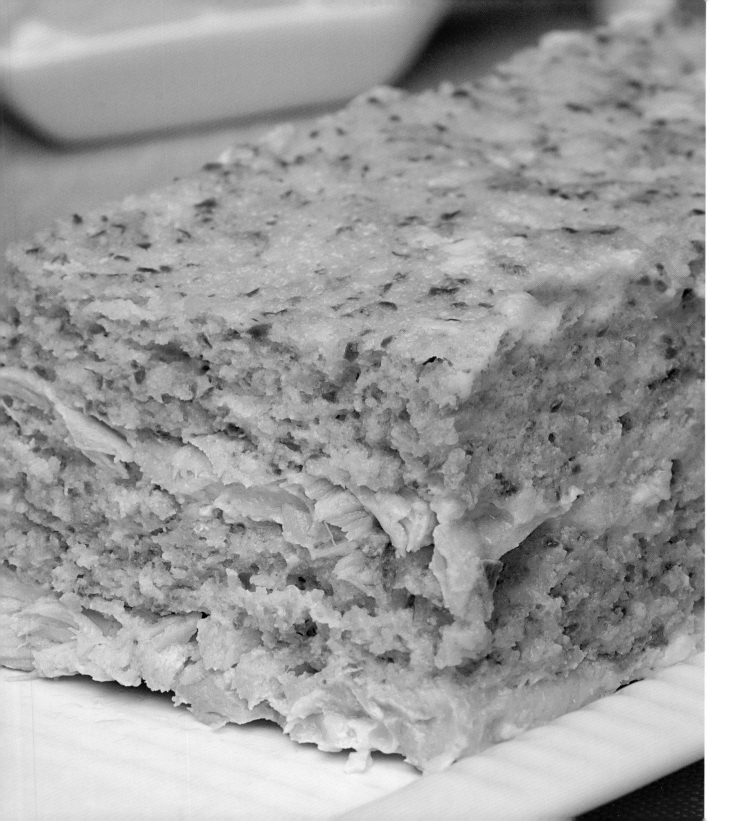

Fish soup with shellfish

Serves 5 to 6

Preparation: 10 minutes
Cooking time: 20 minutes

- 4½ lb (2 kg) assorted fish (monkfish, conger eel, bream, hake, mullet, cod . . .)
- 12 langoustines, tiger prawns, or giant scampi – uncooked
- 1 litre (2 pints) mussels
- 4 white leeks
- 1 stick of celery with leaves removed
- 1 onion
- 3 shallots
- 3 cloves garlic
- 1 bouquet garni
- 3 tablespoons of low fat crème fraîche or soya cream
- Olive oil
- Sea salt, peppercorns, Cayenne pepper

- Have the fish cleaned, de-scaled, and trimmed by the fishmonger. Cut into sections (very large slices). Have the mussels cleaned by the fishmonger.
- Peel, wash, and chop finely the celery, leeks, onion, shallots, and garlic.
- In a large casserole, heat 3 tablespoons of olive oil and sweat the vegetables for 5 minutes.
- Add 1.5 litres (3 pints) water, the bouquet garni, salt, peppercorns, and 3 good pinches of Cayenne pepper. Simmer the soup for 15 to 20 minutes with the lid removed.
- Add the fish to the soup: first, the fish with solid flesh (monkfish, conger eel) and then about 5 minutes later, the fish with fine grained flesh (hake, cod, bream, mullet . . .).
- Add the mussels and the langoustines 2 minutes later and leave to cook for a further 3 to 5 minutes.
- With a slotted spoon, recover the fish and shellfish and keep warm in a soup tureen.
- Remove the bouquet garni from the soup. Adjust the seasoning and add the crème fraîche. Cook for a further 1 or 2 minutes and pour over the fish.
- Serve immediately.

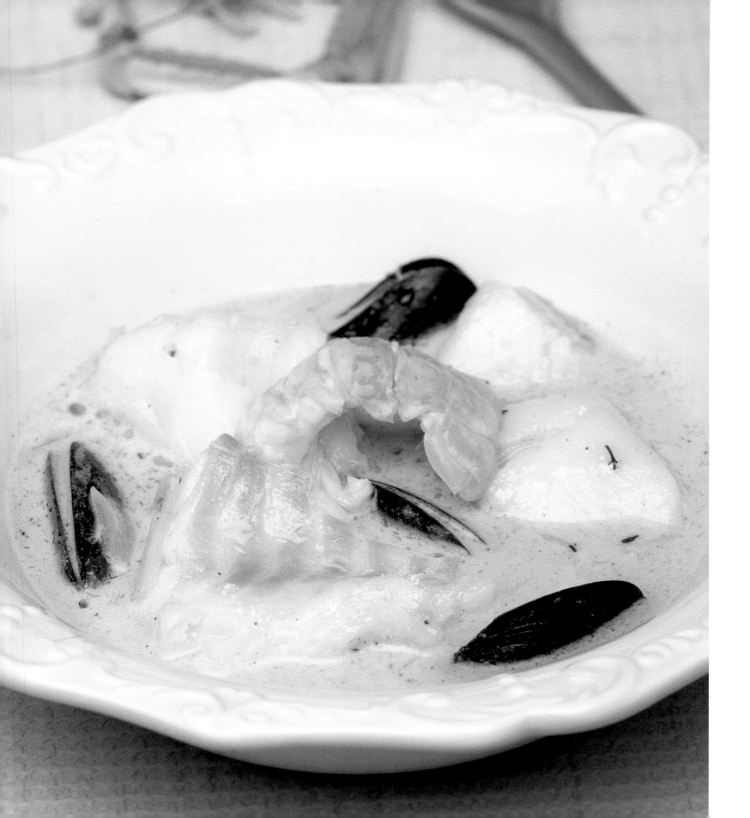

Scallops with raw ham

Serves 4

Preparation: 10 minutes
Cooking time: 25 minutes

- 16 raw scallops
- 1 tablespoon olive oil
- 1 shallot
- 5oz (150 g) raw ham
- 4 tablespoons low-fat crème fraîche
- 1 glass dry white wine
- Salt, pepper

- Fry the chopped shallot in the olive oil.
- Add the scallops and fry for a further 2 minutes only. Season with salt and pepper.
- Add the white wine and the ham, cut into broad strips. Simmer on a low heat for 15 minutes.
- Add the crème fraîche just before serving.

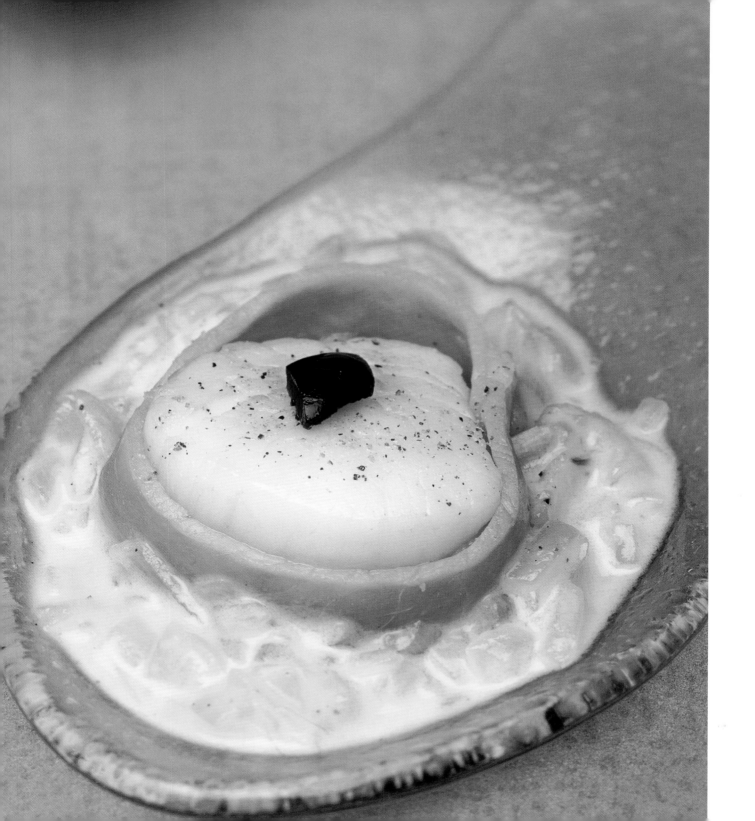

Brown rice paella

Serves 6

Preparation: 1 hour
Cooking time: 1 hour

- 1 large chicken (l.2 kg or 2½ lb), jointed and with ail fat removed
- 18oz (500 g) squid
- 18oz (500 g) scampi
- A dozen large mussels
- 12oz (350 g) long-grain brown rice

- 9oz (250 g) peas
- 26oz (750 g) tinned peeled tomatoes
- 3 good-sized onions
- 4 to 5 tablespoons olive oil
- 1 good pinch saffron
- Salt, pepper

- Soak the brown rice in cold water for 3 hours. Drain and part-cook for 15 minutes.
- In a large pan or paëlla dish, fry the chicken joints in olive oil until they are golden. Remove and set aside.
- In the same pan, fry the chopped onions. Add the tomatoes, chopped and drained.
- Return the chicken to the pan, season with salt and pepper and mingle the ingredients thoroughly.
- Simmer for 30 minutes, adding a little boiling water if necessary.
- Add the squid, cleaned and sliced in rings, together with the peas and the scampi.
- Strew the partly cooked rice into the pan, which should at this stage contain at least 750 ml of liquid.
- Cook for 10 minutes, stirring continuously. Sprinkle with saffron and cook for a further 25 minutes, continuing to stir.
- Wash the mussels, scraping them well, and add them 5 minutes from the end of the cooking time, so that they open up.

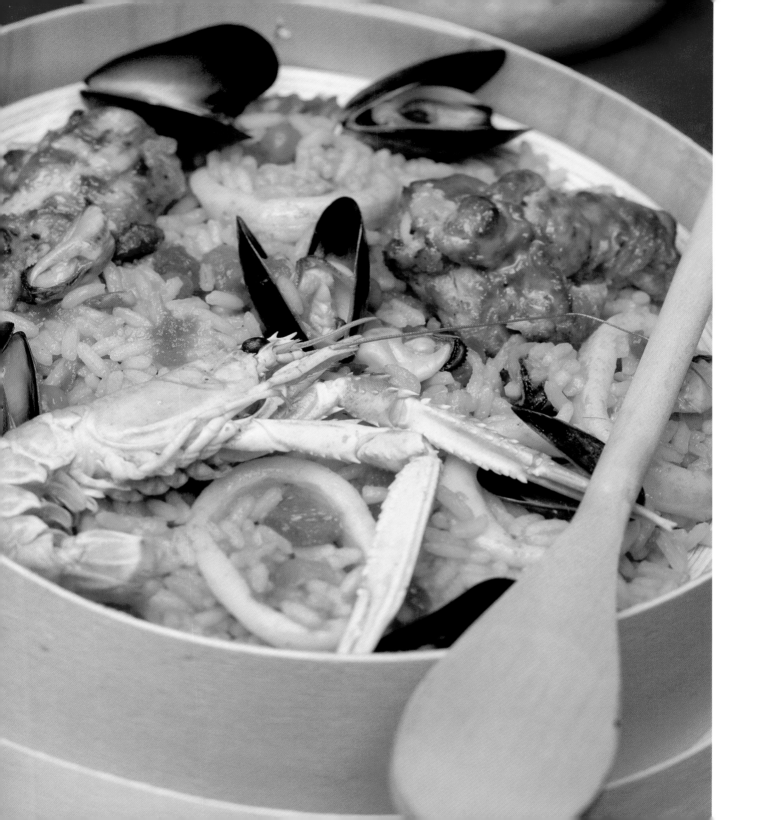

Fish loaf

Serves 6

Preparation: 15 minutes
Cooking time: 40 minutes

- 21oz (600 g) hake fillets
- 2 or 3 ripe tomatoes
- 6 eggs
- 4 cloves garlic
- 1 bunch basil
- 4 tablespoons olive oil
- Salt, pepper

- Plunge the tomatoes into boiling water for 30 seconds, skin and remove the seeds.
- Fry gently with the crushed garlic in the olive oil until all the liquid disappears.
- Blend the raw hake fillets and add the tomato purée, the eggs (lightly beaten), the basil leaves (chopped), salt, and pepper.
- Oil a loaf tin, pour the mixture in and cook in a bain-marie in a moderate oven at 180°C (350°F, gas mark 4) for 40 minutes.
- Turn out and serve tepid or cold, with an olive oil mayonnaise or a tomato coulis.

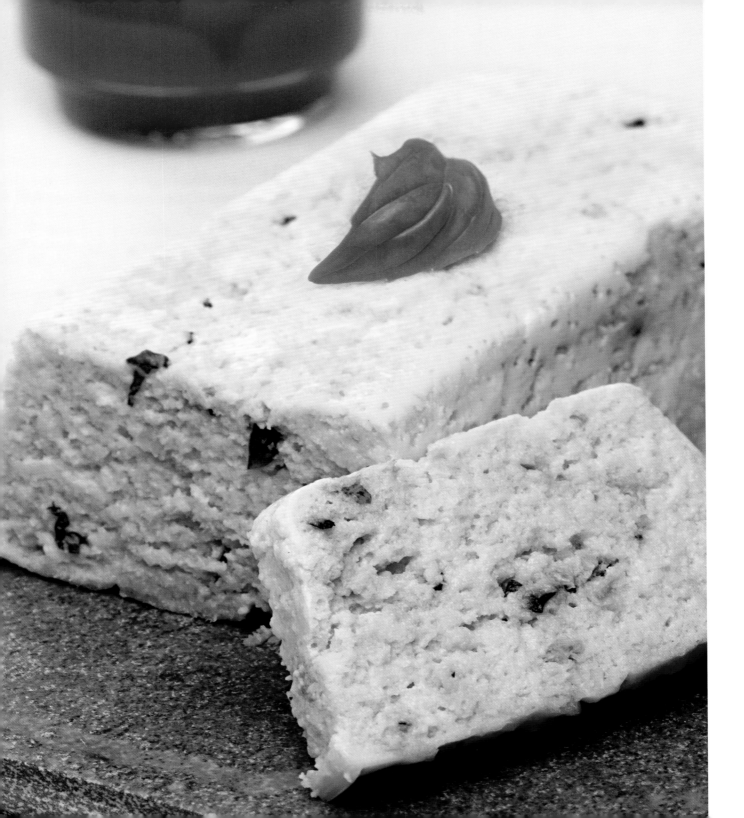

Baked spinach and clams with a cheese topping

Serves 6

Preparation: 20 minutes
Cooking time: 20 minutes

- 4 ½ lb (2 kg) clams
- 2 finely sliced shallots
- 18oz (500 g) spinach
- 3 tablespoons olive oil
- 7oz (200 g) low fat crème fraîche or soya cream
- 2oz (50 g) grated Emmenthal cheese
- Salt, pepper

- Rinse the clams under running water.
- Place over a high heat, together with the shallots, for 5 minutes so that they open up. Remove from their shells.
- Remove the spinach stalks and blanch for 5 minutes in boiling salted water. Drain very thoroughly, chop roughly, and fry in the olive oil, on a high heat, for 5 minutes.
- Mix together the spinach, the clams, and the crème fraîche.
- Pour this mixture into a gratin dish, sprinkle with grated Emmenthal and place in a hot oven at 220°C (425°F, gas mark 7) for 10 minutes.
- Serve hot.

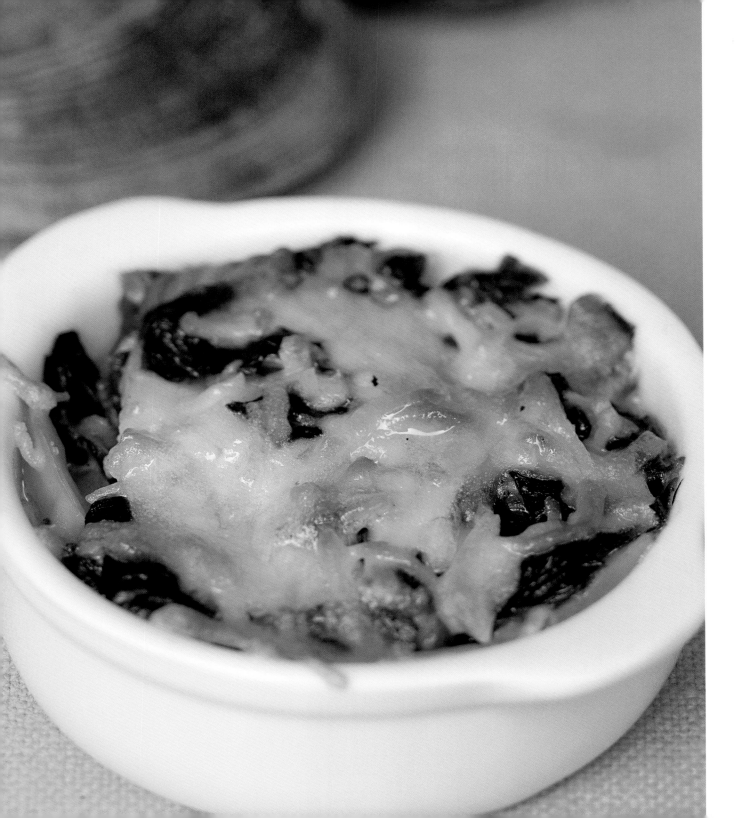

Individual salmon
and mint moulds
Serves 4

Preparation: 1 hour
Cooking time: 20 minutes
Refrigeration: 12 hours

- 1 slice smoked salmon
- 18oz (500 g) fresh salmon fillet
- 2 to 3 tablespoons fresh mint
- 2 leaves (or 2 teaspoons powdered) Gelatine
- 1 tablespoon low-fat crème fraîche
- 1 large courgette
- Olive oil
- Salt, pepper

- Cook the fresh salmon fillet, wrapped in paper or foil parcels, in the oven for 30 minutes or wrap in foil and steam. Allow to cool.
- Wash and chop the fresh mint. Wash the courgette and slice thinly lengthwise, leaving the skin on.
- Fry the courgette slices in olive oil until golden (30 seconds on each side, on a high heat). Leave to cool on kitchen paper.
- Flake the cooked salmon roughly and chop the smoked salmon.
- Soften the gelatine leaves in cold water and drain. Heat the olive oil gently and add the gelatine leaves.
- Combine this liquid with the salmon and add the crème fraîche and mint.
- Mix well together and season with salt and pepper.
- Line 4 ramekins with slices of courgette and pour the mixture in.
- Leave for 12 hours in the refrigerator.
- Remove thirty minutes before serving and turn out at the last minute.

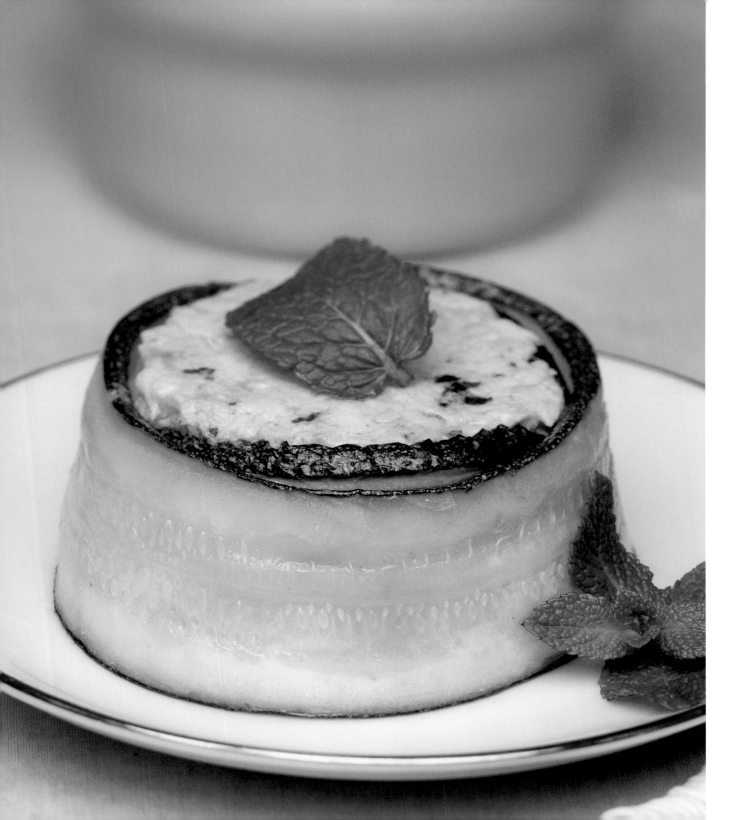

Tuna and olive spread

Serves 4

Preparation: 10 minutes

- 7oz (200 g) tuna in brine
- 4oz (100 g) black olives, pitted
- 2oz (50 g) capers
- 1 tablespoon low-fat crème fraîche
- 2 egg yolks
- 1 clove garlic
- Olive oil
- Salt, pepper, Cayenne pepper

- Drain the tuna. Peel the garlic. Put the tuna, stoned olives, capers, egg yolks, garlic and crème fraîche through the blender.
- Add olive oil gradually until a smooth paste is obtained.
- Taste, add salt if necessary, and season with pepper and Cayenne. Refrigerate.

Suggestions:
The spread can be used to fill celery or chicory leaves for a party buffet, or to garnish small raw tomatoes, hard-boiled egg whites, cooked artichoke bases or mushrooms.

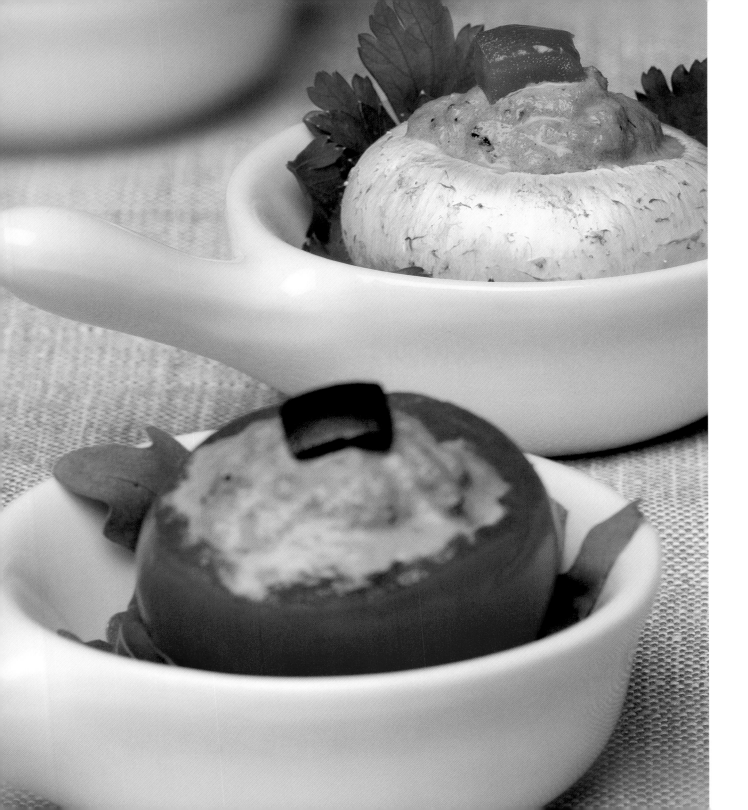

Langoustines with green peppercorns

Serves 4

Preparation: 25 minutes
Cooking time: 20 minutes

- 1lb (500 g) langoustines
- 3 shallots – sliced
- 20 cl (7fl oz) dry white wine
- 2oz (50 g) low fat crème fraîche or soya cream
- Olive oil
- 2 tablespoons green peppercorns

- In a large pot over a low heat, fry the shallots in a tablespoon of olive oil until translucent.
- Add the white wine and simmer for 2 minutes.
- Then add the langoustines and cook over a high heat for 5 minutes.
- Take out the langoustines and reserve on a serving dish.
- Add the peppercorns to the cooking juices and reduce by half.
- Turn down the heat and add the crème fraîche. Cook for 2 minutes. Reserve and keep warm.
- Peel the langoustines. Add the tails to the sauce and heat for 2 to 3 minutes before serving.

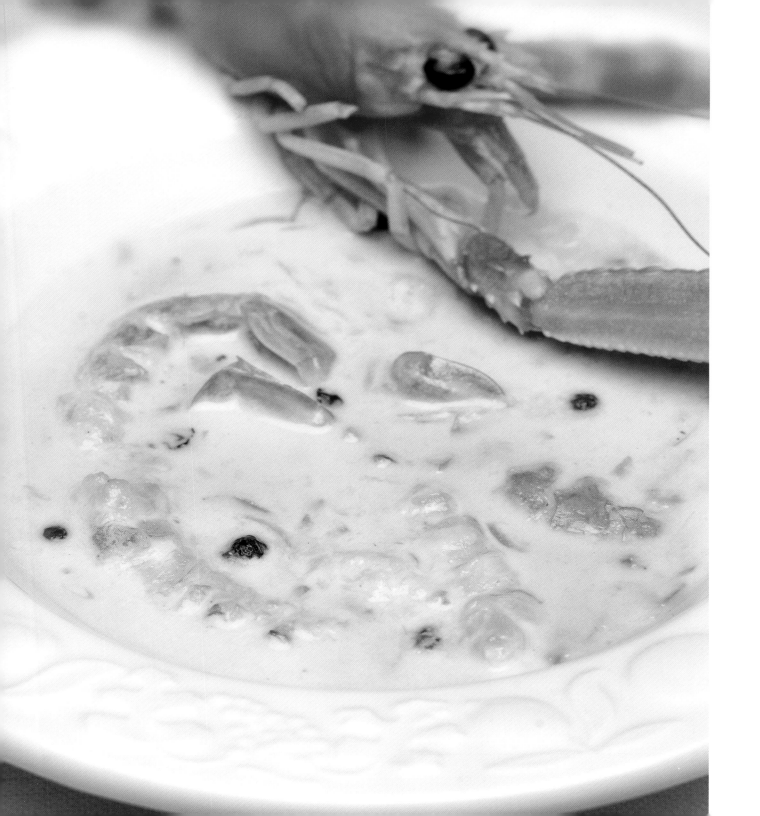

Red mullet with aniseed

Serves 4

Preparation: 15 minutes
Cooking time: 20 minutes

- 4 red mullet, cleaned, de-scaled and pared
- 14oz (400 g) fennel
- 1 teaspoon aniseed grains
- Olive oil
- Salt, freshly ground pepper

- Clean the fennel and cut into strips.
- Blanch in boiling salted water for 6 minutes. Drain well.
- In an ovenproof dish, make a bed of fennel using half the strips. Place the fish on top. Cover with the remainder of the fennel. Sprinkle the aniseed grains over the dish. Sprinkle with olive oil. Season with salt and pepper.
- Place in a very hot oven at 250°C (450°F, gas mark 8) for about 12 minutes.
- Serve in the ovenproof dish.

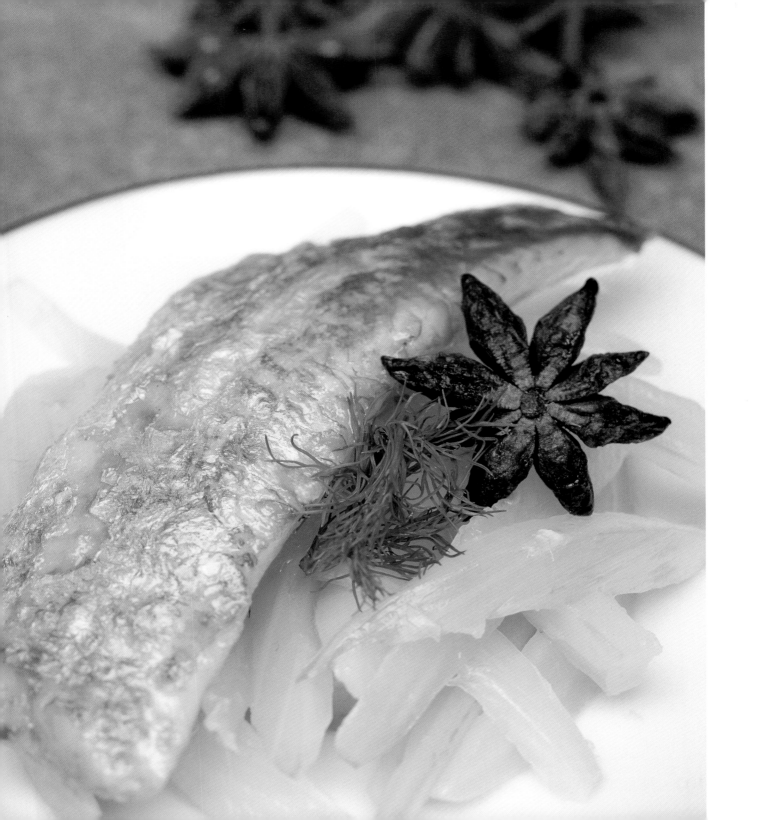

Red mullet with a fresh mint sauce

Serves 4

Preparation: 10 minutes
Cooking time: 15 minutes

- 8 red mullet cleaned and de-scaled
- 4oz (100 g) freshly chopped mint
- 6 cloves garlic
- 2fl oz (5 cl) old wine vinegar
- 2fl oz (5 cl) balsamic vinegar
- 3 tablespoons olive oil
- Salt, freshly ground pepper

- Pre-heat the oven to a very cool at 65°C (140°F).
- Take a non-stick pan, add 2 tablespoons olive oil and cook the red mullet for 4 minutes each side. Season with salt and pepper during the cooking.
- Reserve and keep warm in the oven.
- Slice the garlic very finely.
- Pour the two vinegars and 1 tablespoon olive oil into a pan. Add the garlic and chopped mint. Season lightly with salt and pepper.
- Bring to the boil and stir for 4 to 5 minutes.
- Remove the red mullet from the oven, pour the sauce over the fish, and serve.

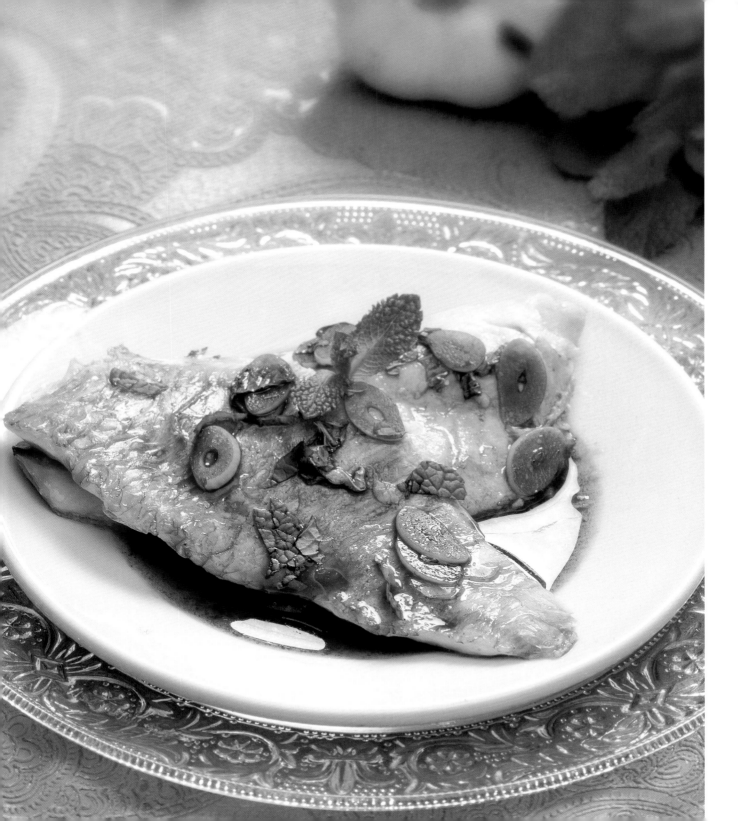

Red mullet with Mediterranean vegetables

Serves 6

Preparation: 35 minutes
Cooking time: 15 minutes

- 6 red mullet (250 g or 9oz each) or 12 fillets
- 11oz (300 g) courgettes
- 11oz (300 g) tomatoes
- 14oz (400 g) aubergines
- 3 cloves garlic
- 1 teaspoon ground coriander
- Thyme, bay leaf
- Olive oil
- 1 lemon
- Tarragon, chervil, parsley, 8 leaves basil
- Salt, pepper
- Court-bouillon, coarse salt

- Wash, scale, and fillet the red mullet. Cook in a court bouillon, uncovered, for 15 minutes. Remove from the court bouillon and place in an ovenproof dish.
- Strain the cooking liquid and pour a little over the fish so it is just covered.
- Cook in a hot oven at 200°C (400°F, gas mark 6) for 5 minutes.
- Slice the tomatoes, courgettes, and aubergines thinly and leave for half an hour covered with coarse salt to draw out the liquid. Arrange on a gratin dish and drizzle a little olive oil over.
- Season with salt and pepper and add the sprig of thyme and the bay leaf, coriander and chopped garlic.
- Roast in a hot oven at 200°C (400°F, gas mark 6) for 15 minutes.
- Remove the thyme and bay leaf. Chop the basil, parsley, tarragon and chervil and mix with 6 tablespoons olive oil and the juice of a lemon. Season with salt and pepper and heat.
- Serve the red mullet fillets surrounded with the vegetables and with the dressing poured over.

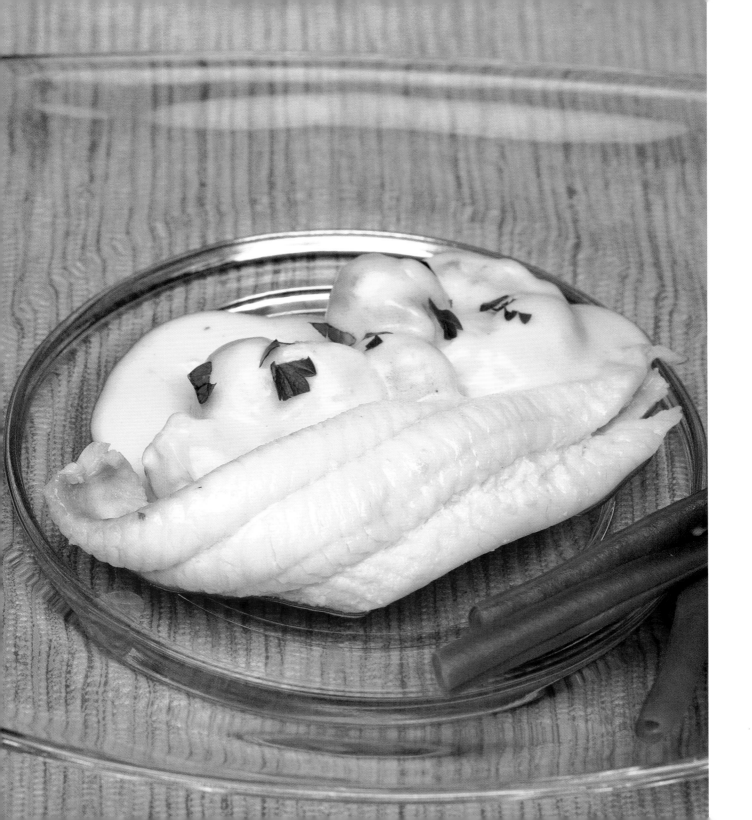

White fish soufflé served with watercress sauce

Serves 6

Preparation: 20 minutes
Cooking time: 25 minutes

- 7oz (200 g) white fish fillets
- 4 eggs
- 6 tablespoons crème fraîche
- Olive oil
- 2 teaspoons lemon juice
- 2 tablespoons chopped fresh parsley

For the sauce:
- 1 bunch watercress
- 6 tablespoons white wine
- 2 tablespoons whipped cream
- 2 shallots
- Salt, pepper

- Clean the fish fillets, washing in cold water and patting dry with absorbent kitchen paper.
- Process, adding the egg yolks and crème fraîche.
- Season with the lemon juice, chopped parsley, salt, and pepper.
- Beat the egg whites until they form stiff peaks and fold them very gently into the mixture so that they do not collapse.
- Oil straight-sided individual moulds and fill with the mixture.
- Cook in an oven set at 180°C (350°F, gas mark 4) for 20 minutes. Turn the oven up to 200°C (400°F, gas mark 6) and cook for a further 5 minutes.
- Meanwhile, prepare the sauce, as follows: Reduce the watercress and shallots in the white wine for a few minutes on a high heat. Put the mixture through a blender and return to the pan to thicken over a low heat.
- Put the mixture through a fine sieve to obtain a smooth sauce. Stir in the whipped cream and season with salt and pepper.
- Serve the soufflés on individual plates accompanied by the sauce.

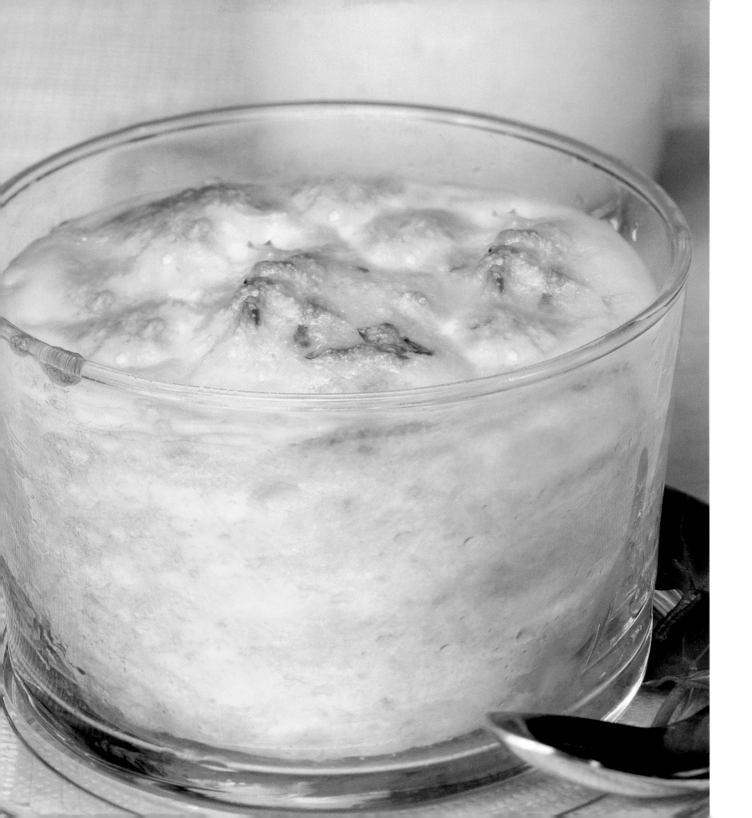

Scallops with shallots and cream of soya   Serves 4

Preparation: 5 minutes
Cooking time: 10 minutes

- 16 scallops
- 8 shallots – sliced
- 5fl oz (15 cl) dry white wine
- 4 tablespoons olive oil
- 7fl oz (20 cl) soya cream
- 2 teaspoons Herbes de Provence
- Salt, freshly ground pepper, Cayenne pepper

- Fry the shallots over a gentle heat, stirring occasionally for 5 minutes till they are translucent.
- Season with salt, pepper, and Cayenne pepper. Sprinkle with Herbes de Provence.
- Add the scallops. Raise the heat slightly and brown for a minute each side. Slowly add the wine. Stir and leave to simmer for 1 minute.
- Add the soya cream. Allow to simmer for a further minute.
- Serve immediately in warm plates.

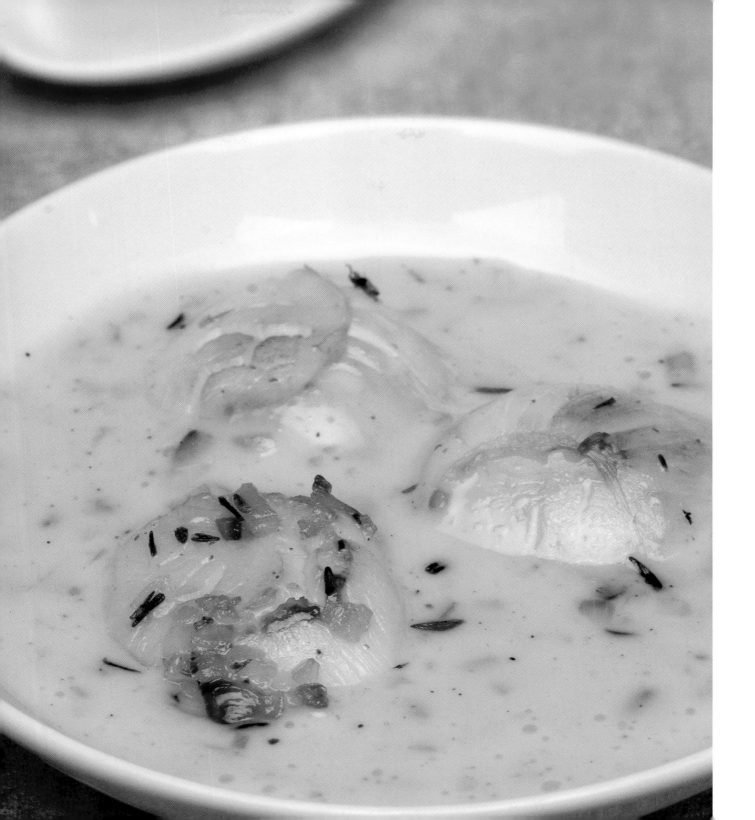

Tuna tartare

Serves 4

Preparation: 20 minutes
Refrigeration: 1 to 2 hours

- 2¼ lb (1 kg) very fresh tuna
- 4 shallots – very finely chopped
- 2 lemons
- 3 tablespoons olive oil
- 1 bunch fresh coriander
- 3 tablespoons freshly chopped parsley
- 1 tablespoon chopped chives
- Salt, freshly ground pepper
- 1 teaspoon Cayenne pepper

- Prepare the tuna by removing the skin and all the bones.
- Cut the flesh into small ½ cm (¼ in) cubes.
- Season with salt, pepper, and Cayenne pepper.
- Pour olive oil over the top and mix well.
- Add the chopped shallots, parsley, chives, and coriander.
- Place in the fridge for 1 or 2 hours.
- Before eating, squeeze the juice of 2 lemons over the dish.

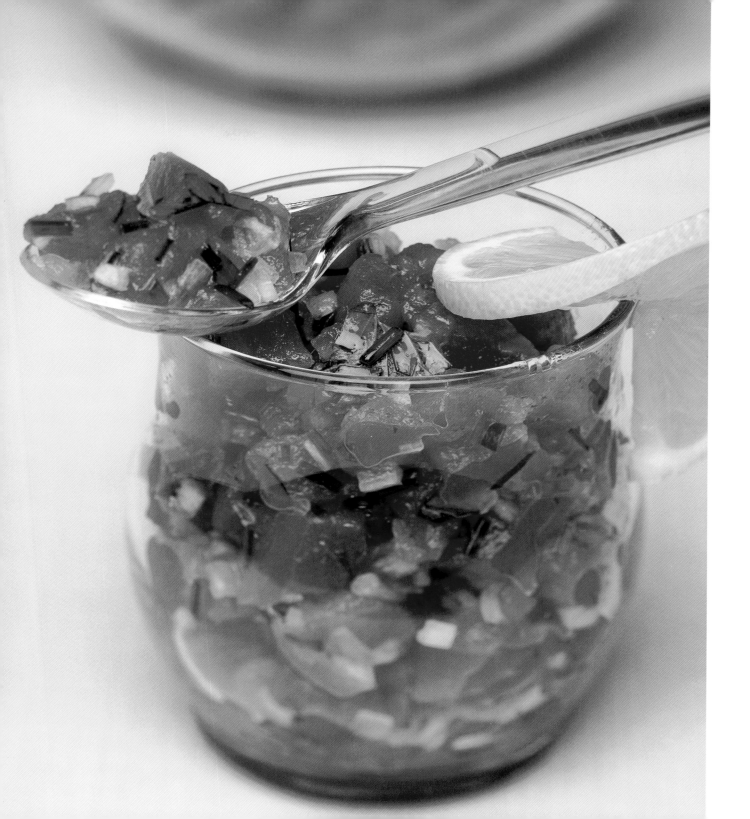

Terrine of salmon trout with a fennel coulis Serves 4

Preparation: 1 hour
Cooking time: 20 minutes
Refrigeration: 12 hours

- 1 small salmon trout (about 1 kg or 2¼ lb)
- 7oz (200 ml) low-fat crème fraîche or soya cream
- 1/4 litre aspic (made from aspic jelly powder)
- 2 sprigs thyme
- 3 bay leaves
- 1 large onion spiked with 3 cloves

- 1 clove garlic
- 21oz (600 g) fennel
- 1 lime
- 2 tablespoons olive oil
- 1 bunch dill
- Salt, peppercorns

- Cook the trout in a court-bouillon, by using the salt, peppercorns, the onion spiked with cloves, bay leaves, thyme, and the clove of garlic in the cooking water.
- From the moment the water boils, allow 10 minutes over a 1ow heat. Remove from the heat and allow trout to cool in the court-bouillon,
- Clean the fennel, removing any stalks which are too tough. .Cut each stalks in two and cook in the pressure cooker for 10 minutes.
- Pour the cooking liquid through a sieve and use it to make the aspic, following the instructions on the packet.
- Skin and bone the fish and break up the flesh with a fork. Allow the aspic to cool slightly before adding half of it to the fish and putting the mixture through the blender. Then add the remainder of the aspic, the cream and salt and pepper to season.
- Moisten a loaf tin, transfer the mixture to it and leave in the refrigerator to set for 12 hours.
- Crush the fennel in the food processor, ad ding the lemon juice.
- Strain the purée through a sieve to make a coulis and season with salt, pepper, and finely chopped dill. Chill.
- Remove the mousse from the refrigerator 15 minutes before serving, turn out at the last minute, and serve in thick slices with the fennel coulis.

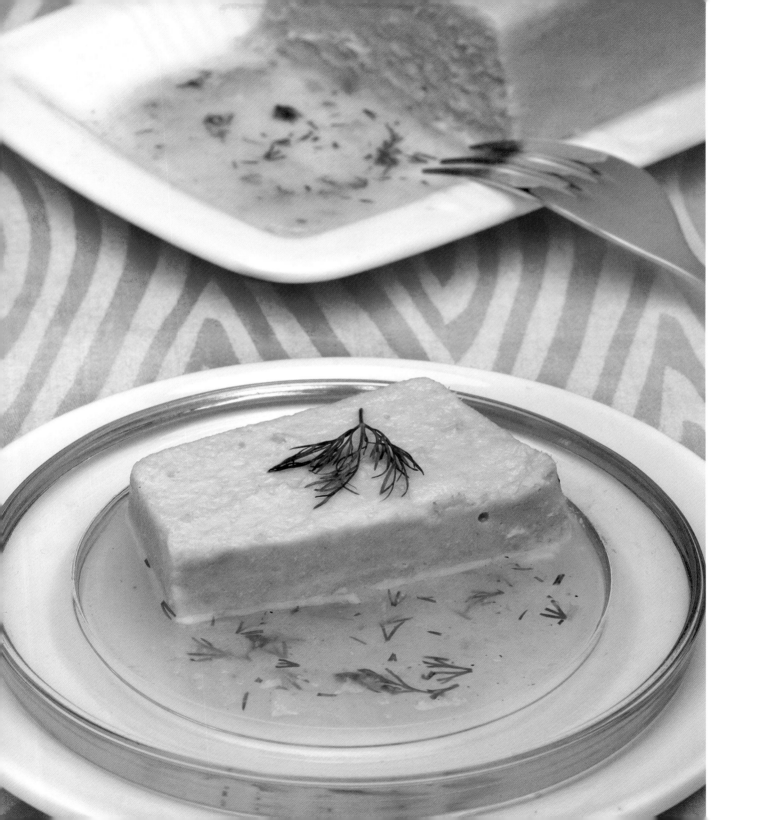

Tuna, tomato and scrambled egg

Serves 4

Preparation: 15 minutes
Cooking time: 45 minutes

- 1lb (500 g) tuna in brine
- 1lb (500 g) tomato coulis
- 3 egg yolks + 1 egg
- 5 cloves garlic – crushed
- 3 tablespoons freshly chopped parsley
- 4 tablespoons olive oil
- 2oz (50 g) gruyère cheese
- 7fl oz (20 cl) low fat whipping cream or soya cream

- Drain the tuna.
- Purée the tuna, garlic, parsley and 4 tablespoons olive oil in a food processor. Reserve.
- Pour the tomato coulis (see below for instructions on how to make a coulis) in a bain-marie with the eggs and cream. Cook, whisking the mixture all the time until it thickens.
- Add the tuna purée and blend with a spatula.
- Put into a soufflé dish and place in a very cool oven at 130°C (Mk.½ – 130°C) for 30 to 35 minutes.
- Before serving, sprinkle with grated gruyère cheese and place under the grill for a few minutes.
- Serve immediately.

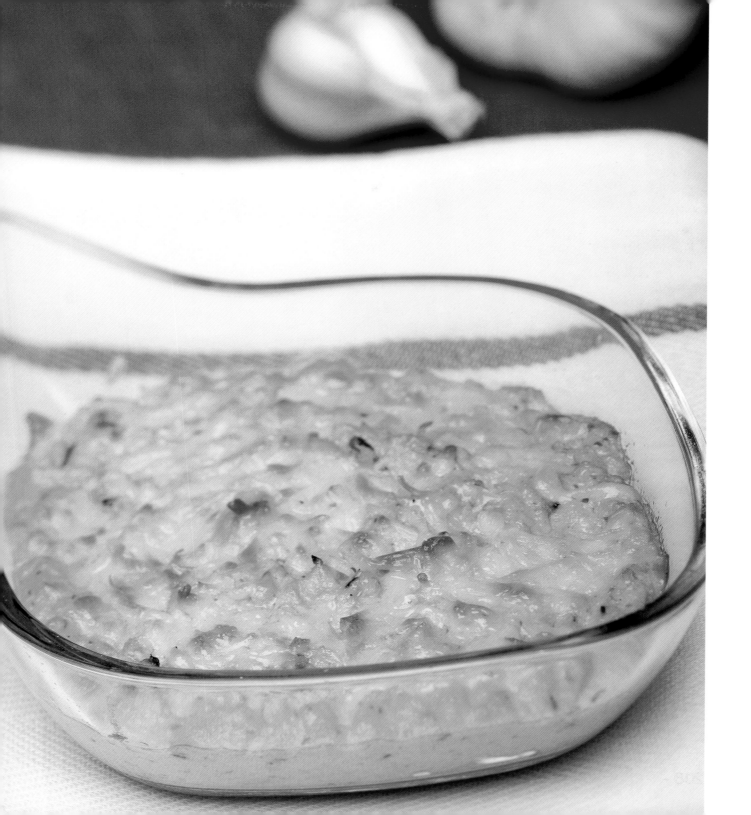

Tuna in aspic

Serves 6

Preparation: 15 minutes
Refrigeration: 6 hours

- 21oz (600 g) tinned tuna in brine
- 1 sachet aspic jelly powder
- 6 to 8 bay leaves
- 1 bunch parsley
- 1 bunch chives
- 7oz (200 g) small button mushrooms, fresh
- 9oz (250 g) fromage frais
- Juice of 1 lemon
- 1 sprig fresh fennel
- Olive oil
- Salt, pepper

- Make the aspic according to the instructions on the packet and pour a little into a savarin mould.
- Lay the bay leaves on the aspic and place in the refrigerator to set.
- Drain and flake the tuna. Place it in the mould, on top of the bay leaves.
- Add the parsley and chives, chopped, and the rest of the aspic. Leave in the refrigerator to set for 6 hours.
- Trim the mushrooms as necessary.
- Wash and season with olive oil, lemon juice, salt, and pepper.
- Make a dressing to accompany the dish, by mixing the fromage frais with lemon juice, chopped fennel, salt, and pepper.
- Turn out the tuna in aspic onto a serving dish, place the mushrooms in the centre and serve with the sauce.

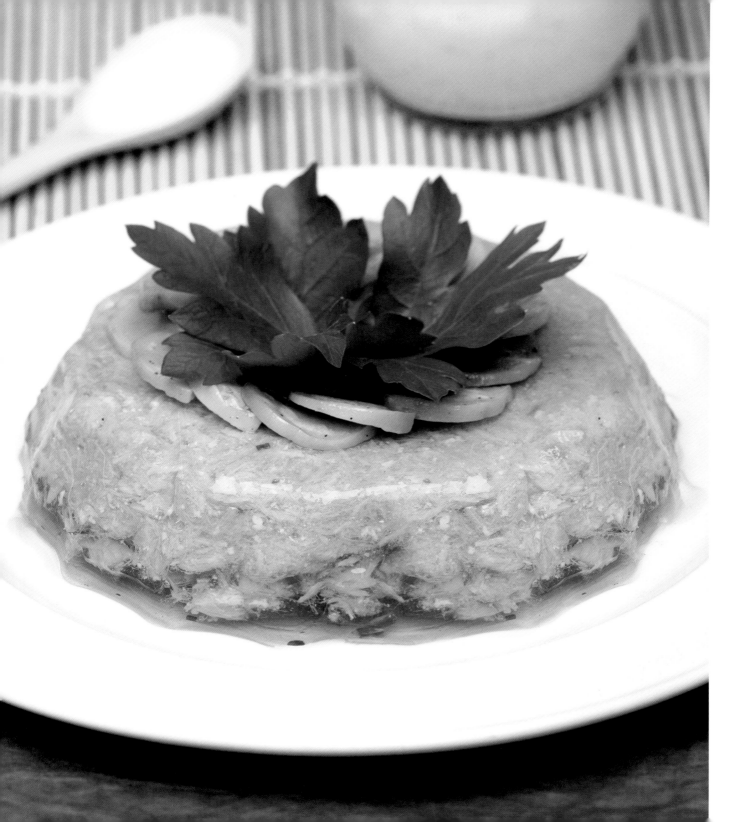

Grilled tuna with bacon

Serves 6

Preparation: 5 minutes
Cooking time: 30 minutes

- 1 tuna fillet of 1.2 kg (2½ lb)
- 12 thin rashers smoked bacon
- 1 tablespoon olive oil

- Salt, pepper
- Roll the tuna up in the bacon rashers and secure with string (rather like a giant tournedos).
- Brush with olive oil on both sides and season with salt and pepper.
- Cook under a hot grill for 15 minutes on each side. Serve at once.

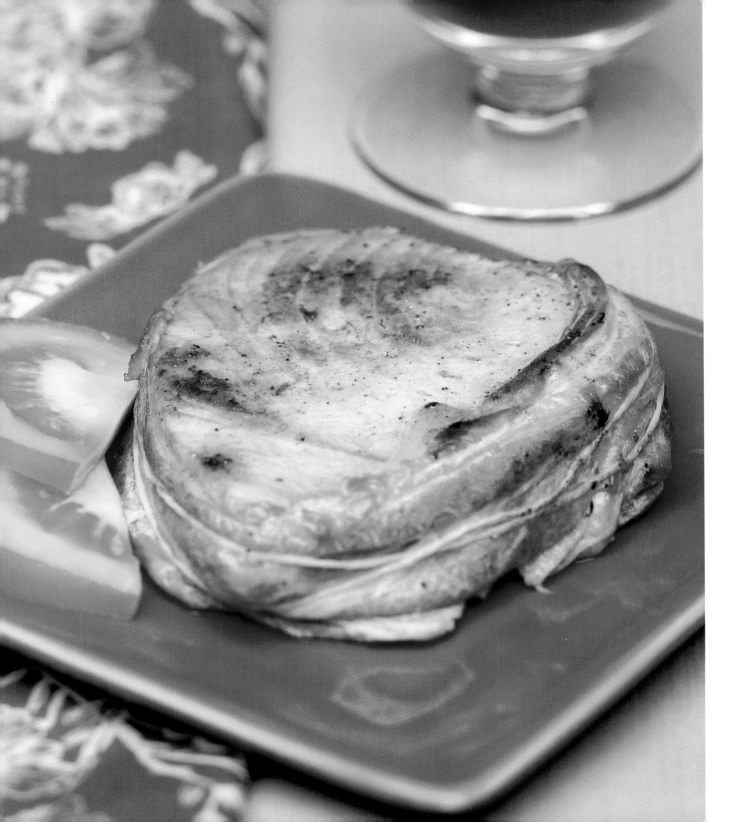

Trout with melted cheese topping

Serves 4

Preparation: 15 minutes
Cooking time: 25 minutes

- 4 trout (9-11oz or 250-300 g each)
- 8 (5 mm thick) slices tomme de Savoie or Emmental
- 1 small tin skinned tomatoes
- 2oz (50 ml) olive oil
- 1 clove garlic
- 4oz (100 g) onions
- 1oz (20 g) basil
- 2oz (50 g) parsley
- Salt, pepper

- Peel the garlic and onion and chop finely.
- Put the tomatoes through the blender. Fry the garlic, onion, and tomatoes in olive oil on a high heat for a few minutes. Season with salt and pepper.
- Clean the trout and place in an ovenproof dish. Pour the tomato sauce over, cover with a sheet of cooking foil and place in the oven at 200°C (400°F, gas mark 6) for 25 minutes.
- 10 minutes from the end of the cooking time, place two slices of cheese on top of each trout.
- Serve decorated with chopped parsley and basil.

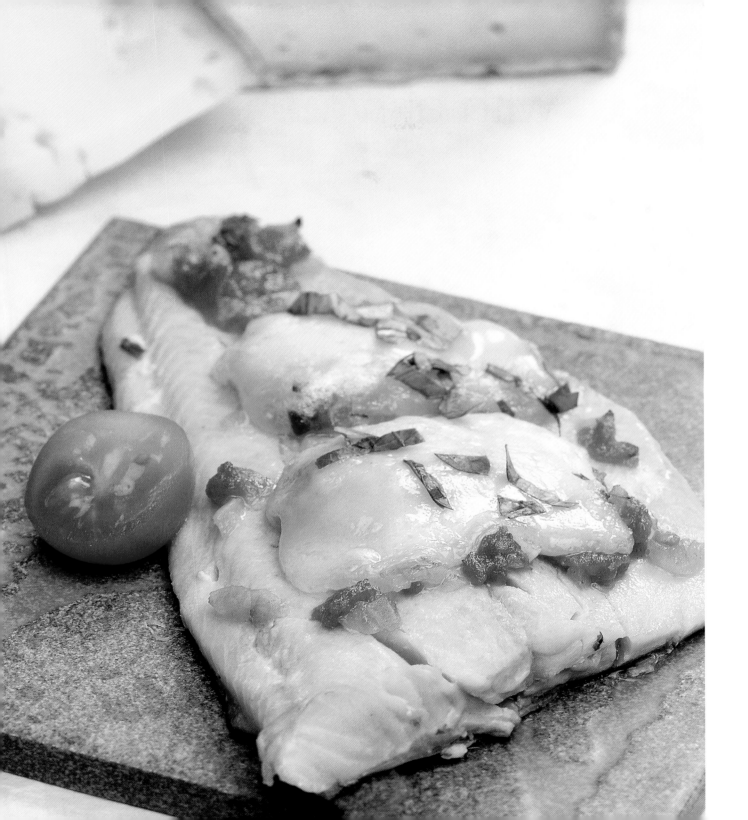

Trout with almonds

Serves 4

Preparation: 10 minutes
Cooking time: 15 minutes

- 4 plump trout
- 3oz (80 g) flaked almonds
- 2 lemons
- 1 tablespoon sherry vinegar
- 2 tablespoons freshly chopped parsley
- Olive oil
- Herbes de Provence
- Salt, freshly ground pepper

- Have the trout cleaned by the fishmonger. Dust the body cavity with Herbes de Provence. Season with salt and pepper.
- In a non-stick frying pan, gently heat 4 tablespoons of olive oil.
- Place the trout in the pan and cook for 6 minutes on each side. Reserve and keep warm on a serving dish in a very cool oven at 80–100°C.
- In another pan, add 1 tablespoon of olive oil and fry the almonds until golden brown. Season with salt and pepper. Add the sherry vinegar.
- Pour the vinegar and almond mixture over the trout.
- Serve with lemons cut in half.

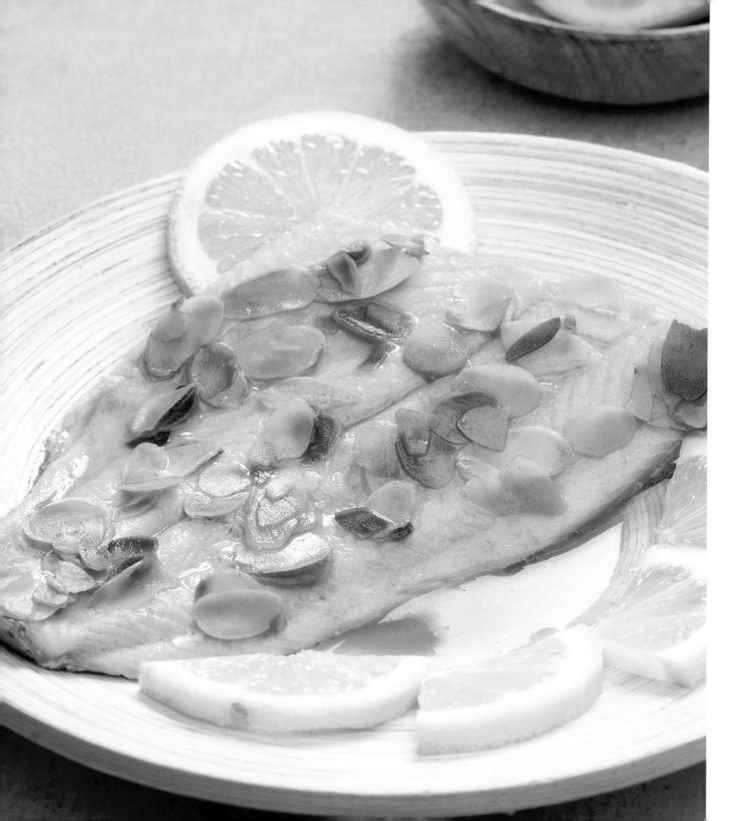

Turbot with sorrel

Serves 4

Preparation: 20 minutes
Cooking time: 40 minutes

- 4 turbot fillets
- 4oz (100 g) sorrel
- 4oz (100 g) low fat crème fraîche or soya cream
- 9fl oz (25 cl) dry white wine
- 9fl oz (25 cl)) fish stock
- 2 egg yolks
- 2 bay leaves – crumbled
- Olive oil
- Salt, pepper

- Wash the fillets under the tap. Dab dry with absorbent kitchen paper.
- Coat an oven dish with olive oil and arrange the fillets on it. Season with salt and pepper. Add the bay leaves. Pour the wine over the top.
- Cook for 20 minutes in a fairly hot oven at 190°C (380°F, gas mark 5). Reserve and keep warm.
- In the meantime, select the best leaves of the sorrel and remove the fibrous stalks. Brown over a very low heat in a pan with a little olive oil.
- Reduce the fish stock by half. Then in a bain-marie, beat the stock, crème fraîche and egg yolks with a whisk.
- Lay a bed of sorrel on the bottom of the serving dish. Place the fillets on top and coat with the sauce.

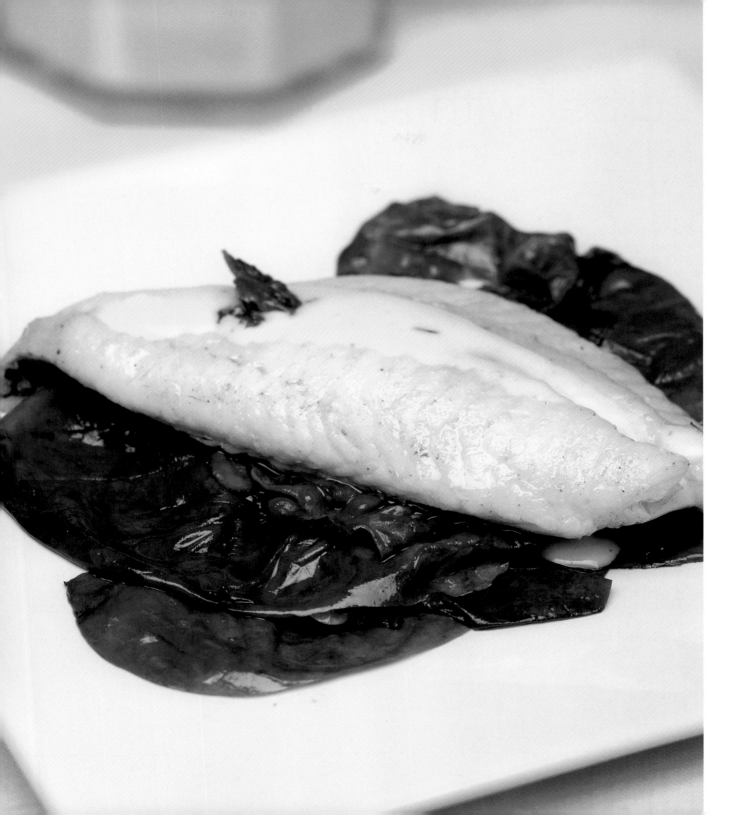

Turbot with fennel

Serves 4

Preparation: 25 minutes
Cooking time: 25 minutes

- 4 turbot fillets weighing together about 800 g (1¾ lb)
- 6 good-sized tomatoes
- 1 bulb fennel
- Juice of 4 lemons
- 10fl oz (30 cl) fish stock
- 4 finely sliced shallots
- 1 clove garlic – crushed
- 2oz (50 g) low fat crème fraîche or soya cream
- Olive oil
- Salt, pepper, thyme

- Wash the fillets under the tap. Dab dry with absorbent kitchen paper.
- Wash the fennel. Cut into fine strips.
- Drop the tomatoes in boiling water for 1 minute, peel and deseed. Cut the flesh into strips.
- In a medium-sized casserole, heat the lemon juice and fish stock. Season with salt and pepper. Add the thyme. Poach the turbot fillets in the liquid for 7 minutes. Reserve and keep warm.
- Reduce the liquid by a quarter, then add the crème fraîche.
- Meanwhile, Brown the fennel, garlic and shallots in a casserole with olive oil. Then cover and sweat a few minutes.
- Add the tomatoes at the last moment to the garlic and shallots.
- Arrange the vegetables on the serving dish. Then lay out the fillets and coat with the sauce.

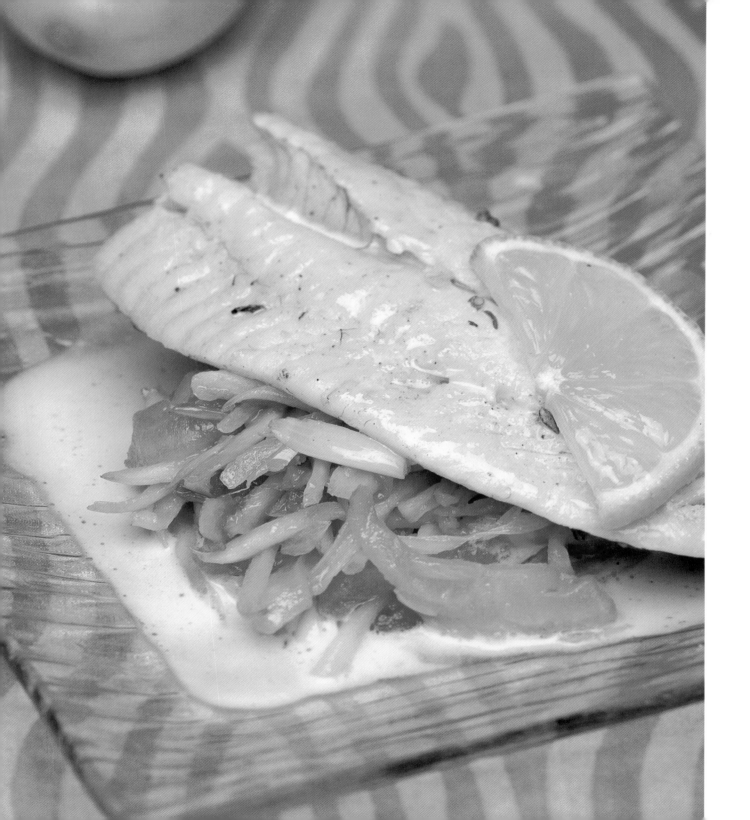

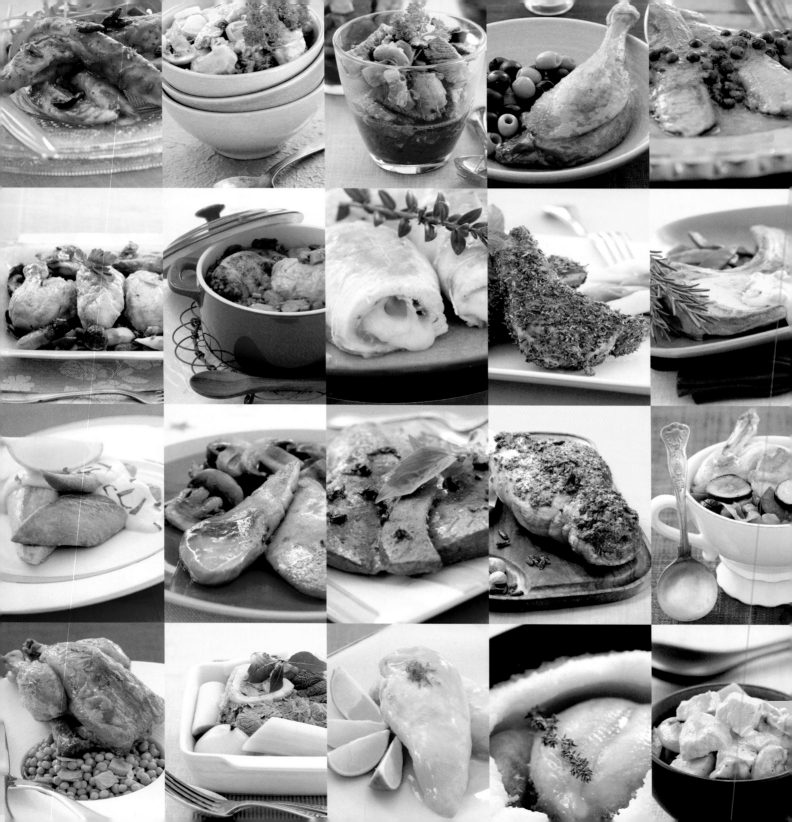

Meat recipes

Chicken breasts in creamy garlic sauce

Serves 4

Preparation: 20 minutes
Cooking time: 1 hour

- 4 boneless chicken breasts
- 2 heads garlic
- 11oz (30 cl) soya cream
- Goose fat
- Salt, freshly ground pepper, mild paprika
- Cayenne pepper
- 1 bunch parsley

- Break up the heads of garlic, peel the cloves, and cook in a steamer for 30 minutes.
- Place the chicken breasts in an ovenware dish and brush with goose fat.
Season with salt, pepper, and sprinkle lightly with Cayenne pepper.
- Put in the oven at 190°C (375°F, gas mark 5) for 20 to 25 minutes.
- Liquidize the garlic cloves with the soya cream. Season with salt, pepper and add the equivalent of ½ teaspoon of mild paprika.
- Remove the chicken breasts from the oven and cut widthways in 1 to 2cm (½ in) slices.
- Rearrange in the cooking dish.
- Coat with the garlic cream and leave in a lukewarm oven at 100°C (200°F, gas mark ½) for 10 to 15 minutes.
- Sprinkle with chopped parsley and serve.

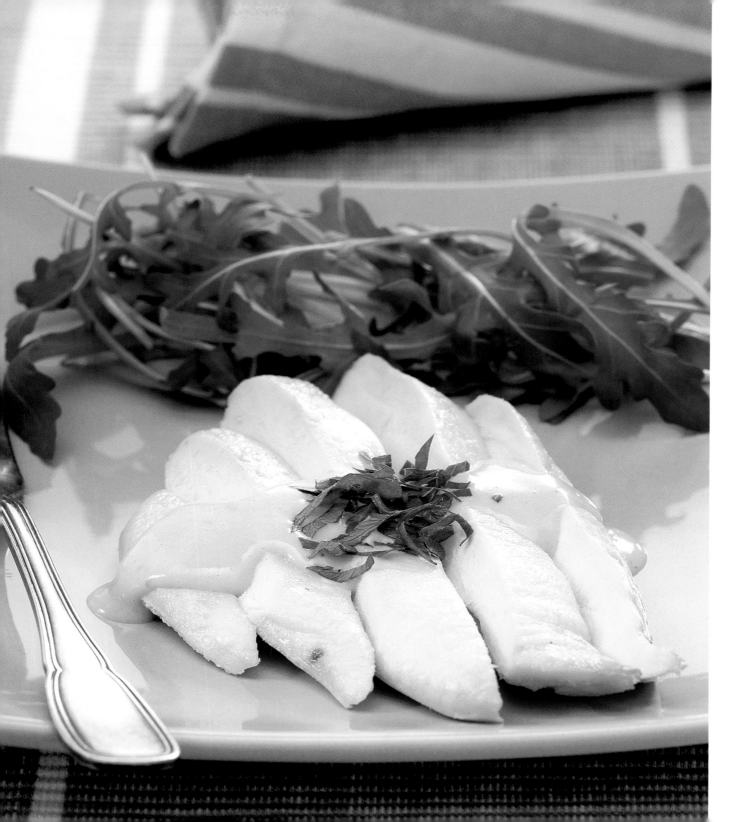

Chicken breasts
with lime Serves 4

Preparation: 15 minutes
Cooking time: 45 minutes

- 4 boneless chicken breasts
- 5 garlic cloves – crushed
- 3 limes
- 4 tablespoons olive oil
- Salt, freshly ground pepper, Cayenne pepper

- In a bowl, make a marinade of lime juice, olive oil, crushed garlic, salt, and pepper. Mix well.
- Dust the chicken breasts lightly with Cayenne pepper and immerse in the marinade.
- Place in the fridge for a few hours, turning from time to time.
- Drain the chicken breasts and put them in a roasting tin. Place in a preheated oven at 190°C (375°F, gas mark 5) and cook for 30 minutes.
- In the meantime, pour the marinade into a pan, bring to the boil and reduce to obtain a thick sauce.
- Serve the chicken breasts coated with this sauce.

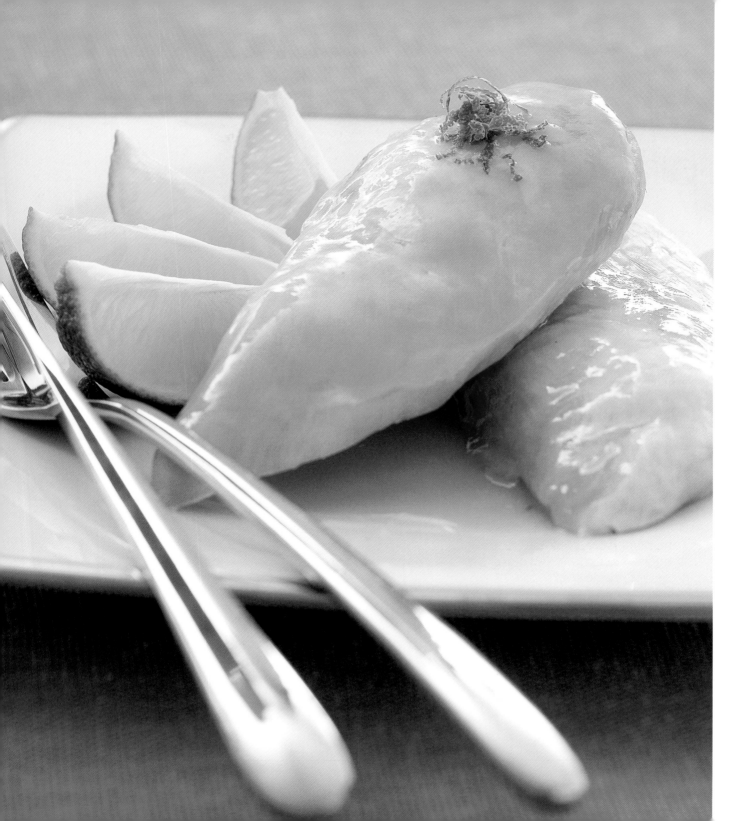

Chicken breasts provençale Serves 4

Preparation: 10 minutes
Cooking time: 15 minutes

- 4 boneless chicken breasts
- 18oz (500 g) fresh tomato purée (or 9oz (250 g) tomato paste + 9fl oz (25 cl) water)
- 1 tablespoon Herbes de Provence
- 4 tablespoons olive oil
- 4 cloves garlic crushed
- Salt, pepper, Cayenne pepper

- Cut the chicken breasts into slices 2cm (1in) thick. Salt and sprinkle with Cayenne pepper.
- Cook in a steamer for 5 minutes.
- Meanwhile, pour the tomato purée into a casserole. Add the crushed garlic, the Herbes de Provence and the 4 tablespoons of olive oil. Salt and pepper.
Stir and put back on a very gentle heat.
- Turn the chicken breasts (with pink centres) into the casserole. Stir well, cover and cook over an extremely low heat for 5 minutes with the lid on. Correct the seasoning before serving.
- If desired, trickle a little olive oil over the chicken when served.

Suggestion :
This dish can be prepared in advance and gently re-heated with the lid on.

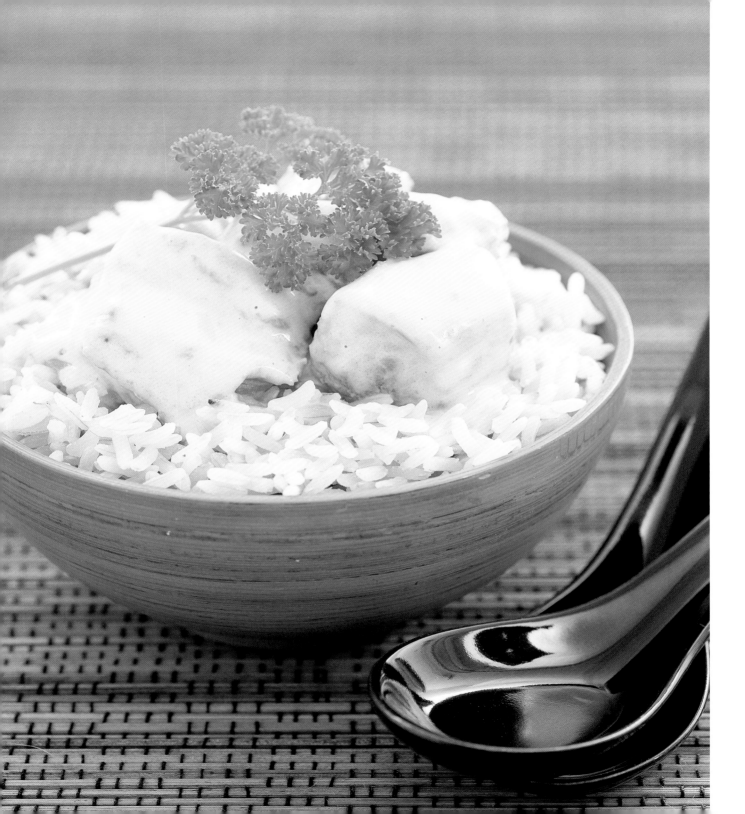

Beef casserole provençale

Serves 5

Preparation: 15 minutes
Cooking time: 2 hours 50 minutes

- 3,3lb (1,5 kg) braising steak or chuck steak cut into cubes
- 5oz (200 g) streaky bacon – diced
- 11oz (300 g) mushrooms
- 9oz (25 cl) red wine with a high tannin content (Corbières, Côtes du Rhône…)
- 10 small onions
- 9oz (25 cl) meat stock
- 1 bouquet garni
- 1 bunch parsley
- Goose fat
- Salt, pepper

- Fry the diced streaky bacon in a non-stick pan over a low heat. Add the onions and heat gently until golden brown. Remove from pan and set aside.
- In a casserole, heat 3 tablespoons of goose fat. On a low heat fry the pieces of meat and brown all over. Pour the stock.
- Add the diced streaky bacon and the onions to casserole. Pour the red wine, season with salt and pepper. Add the bouquet garni. Cover and allow to cook gently for two hours.
- In a saucepan, cook the sliced mushrooms in a tablespoon of the cooking fluid for 15 minutes.
- Remove half of the mushrooms and put them into a blender to make a purée. Add to casserole.
- Remove the cover and cook for a further 30 minutes. Remove the bouquet garni and correct the seasoning. Sprinkle with chopped parsley and serve.

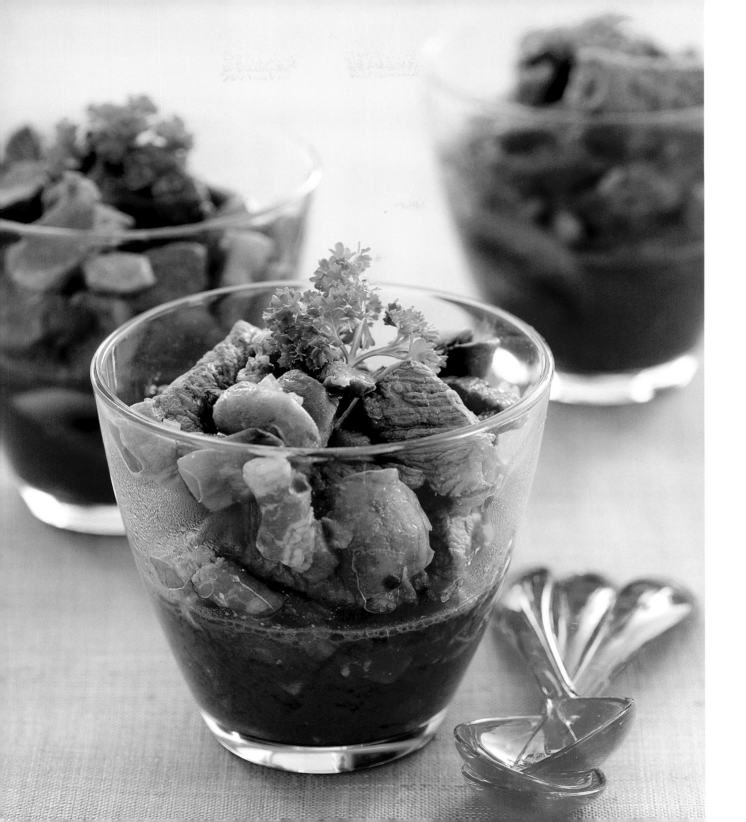

Duck with olives

Serves 4

Preparation: 20 minutes
Cooking time: 2 hours 10 minutes

- 1 large duck with the liver
- 11oz (300 g) green olives – stoned
- 11oz (300 g) black olives – stoned
- 2 eggs
- 2 slices wholemeal bread
- 4fl oz (10 cl) double cream
- 1 onion – peeled
- Salt, freshly ground pepper, Cayenne pepper
- Herbes de Provence
- Olive oil

- Cut up the liver and brown quickly in some olive oil.
- Soak the bread in the double cream and allow to swell.
- Use the liquidizer to make a paste of the liver, a third of the green and black olives, the eggs, and the bread soaked in cream. Season with salt, Herbes de Provence, pepper and Cayenne pepper.
- Stuff the duck with this mixture and seal the body cavity with the onion.
- Put the duck in a roasting tin. Sprinkle salt, pepper and Cayenne pepper over the top and place in the oven at 160°C (320°F, gas mark 2 ½).
- After an hour, slowly pour a glass of salted water over the duck and then add the rest of the olives to the contents of the tin and stir together.
- Return the duck to the oven and continue cooking at a reduced temperature at 130°C (260°F, gas mark ½) for another hour.
- Remove the olives with a slotted spoon and reserve in a warm place. Skim off some of the fat in the tin and deglaze the remainder with a glassful of boiling water.
- Carve the duck in the roasting tin, to conserve the juices. Arrange the pieces on a warm dish.
- Finish deglazing the roasting tin and reheat the sauce before pouring into a warm sauceboat.

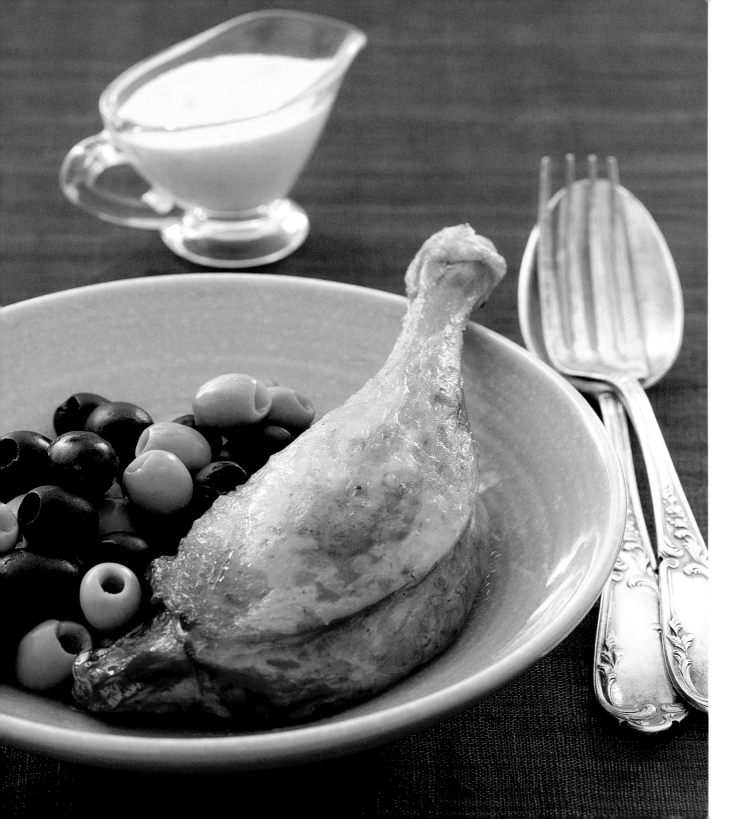

Rack of lamb provençale

Serves 4

Preparation: 25 minutes
Cooking time: 45 minutes

- 1 rack of lamb, weighing about 1kg (2¼ lb)
(8 good-size chops)
- 4fl oz (10 cl) dry white wine
- 5fl oz (15 cl) low fat crème fraîche (or soya cream)
- 1 tablespoon cognac
- 5 cloves garlic – peeled

- Olive oil
- Herbes de Provence
- 14oz (400 g) button mushrooms
- Salt, freshly ground pepper, Cayenne pepper
- 1 tablespoon of chopped parsley

- Cut 2 cloves of garlic into a total of 8 slices. Make deep gashes in the rack of lamb (between each chop) and insert the slivers of garlic.
- Coat the cooking tin with olive oil. Mix 4 tablespoons of olive oil together with salt, pepper and a pinch of Cayenne pepper. Place the rack of lamb in the tin and brush with the seasoned olive oil. Sprinkle with the Herbes de Provence and place in a very hot oven at 250°C (460°F, gas mark 8). Cook for 20 to 25 minutes.
- In the meantime, clean the mushrooms and remove the stalks. Cut into slices – the stalks down their length.
- Brown the mushrooms over a very gentle heat, in a pan with olive oil. Season with salt and pepper. After a few minutes, remove the cooking juices and water they have produced.
- Crush the 3 remaining cloves of garlic and mix them with the parsley. Add them to the mushrooms in the olive oil. Continue cooking over a gentle heat for several minutes, stirring well.
- Take the rack of lamb out of the oven and cut it up in the cooking tin. Reserve the chops and keep warm. Deglaze the tin with the white wine and cognac that have already been heated. Add the crème fraîche and pour into a warm sauceboat.
- Serve the rack on a warm plate surrounded with mushrooms.

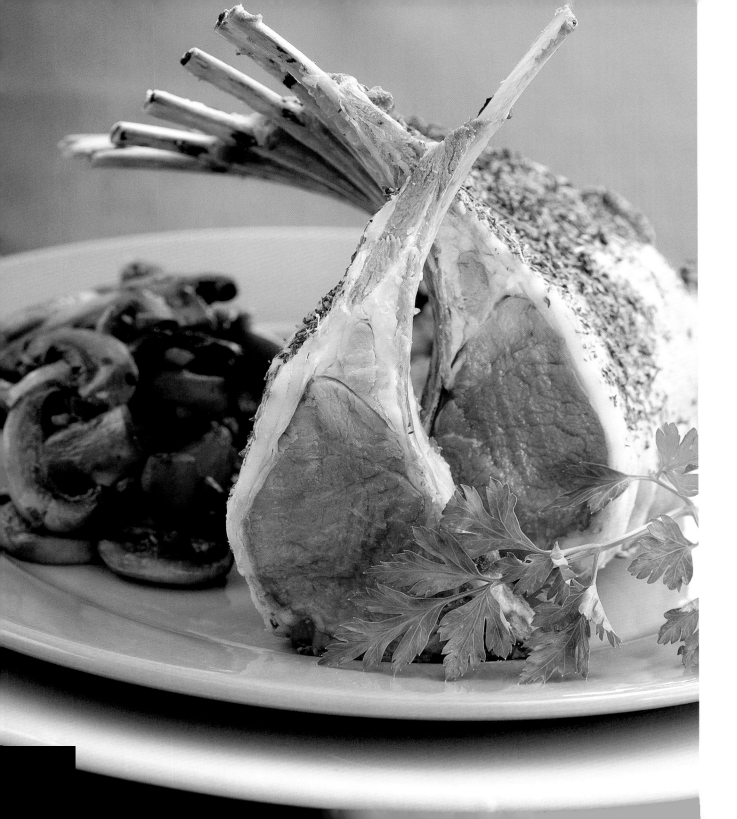

Chili con carne

Serves 6

Preparation: 30 minutes
Cooking time: 3 hours

- 2¼ lb (1 kg) minced beef
- 11oz (300 g) red kidney beans
- 3 onions
- 1 green pepper
- 2 claves garlic
- 1 kg tinned tomatoes

- Salt
- 4oz (100 ml) olive ail
- 2 Cayenne (finger) peppers
- 1 teaspoon ground cumin
- 1 pint, (½ litre) chicken stock
- 1 teaspoon paprika

- Soak the red kidney beans in cold water for 12 hours. Drain, cover with cold water, bring to the boil and cook on a medium heat for 1 ½ hours. Half-way through cooking, add salt and skim. When the beans are done, drain and set on one side.
- On a high heat, fry the minced beef in a casserole in 3 tablespoons olive oil. Season with salt and paprika. Simmer for 10 minutes. Remove the meat and set on one side.
- Wash and dice the green pepper and fry on a low heat in the casserole in 2 tablespoons olive oil. Add the sliced onions and the crushed garlic. When the onions are translucent, add the Cayenne peppers and the cumin.
- Return the meat to the casserole and pour in the chicken stock. Add the tomatoes and mingle the ingredients together.
- Cover and cook on a low heat for 40 minutes. Then add the red kidney beans and replace over a low heat to cook, uncovered, for a further 30 minutes.
- Add more stock during cooking if necessary.
- Serve hot.

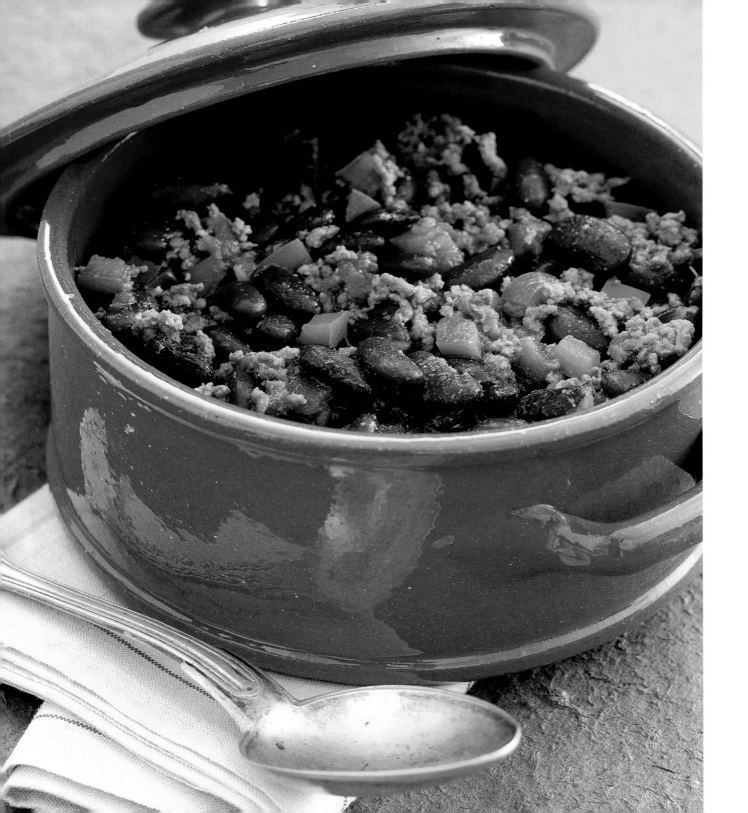

Duck confit
with sauerkraut   Serves 4

Preparation: 10 minutes
Cooking time: 30 minutes

- 4 legs confit of duck
- 21oz (600 g) fresh sauerkraut

- Cut the fat of the confit and put the legs in the top of a steamer.
- Put the sauerkraut in the bottom. Season if necessary.
- Cook for 30 minutes from boiling point.
- Ensure the sauerkraut stays evenly cooked.
- Serve the confit surrounded by the sauerkraut.

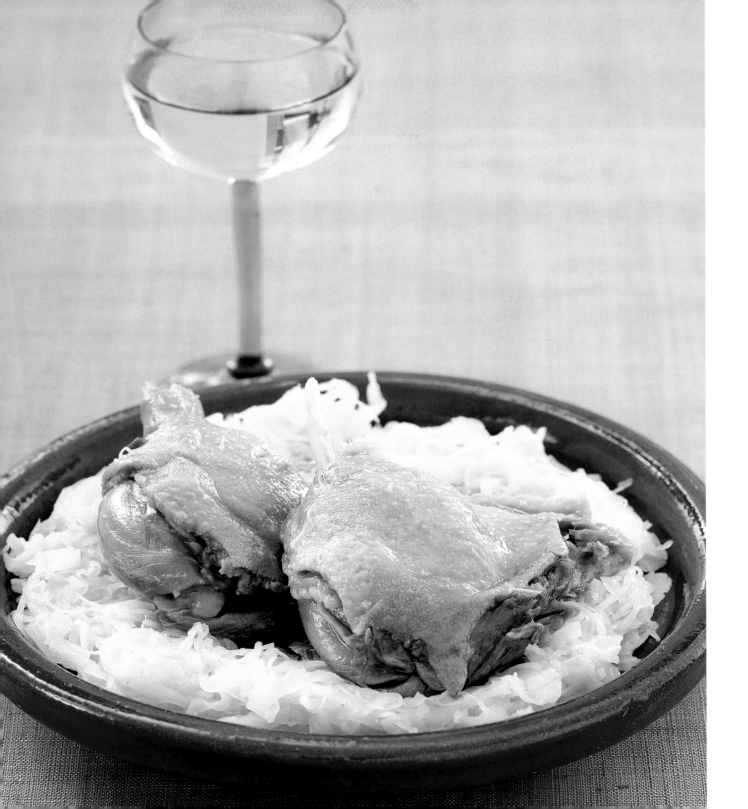

Chicken casserole in wine

Serves 4

Preparation: 30 minutes
Cooking time: 1 hour 10 minutes

- 1 large free-range chicken
- 2 onions – chopped
- 2 cloves garlic
- 4oz (100 g) diced streaky bacon
- 14oz (400 g) tinned mushrooms
- 18fl oz (50 cl) red wine with a high tannin content (Corbières, Madiran, Côtes du Rhône…)
- 2 tablespoons goose fat
- Salt, freshly ground pepper, Cayenne pepper

- Cut the chicken up into several pieces and remove most of the skin.
- Melt the goose fat in a casserole. Lightly brown the onions and garlic over a gentle heat.
- In the meantime, brown the diced streaky bacon in a non-stick pan until most of the fat has melted.
- Fry the chicken pieces in the casserole until golden brown. Add the streaky bacon without the melted fat and add a little red wine. Season with salt, pepper, and Cayenne pepper.
Raise the temperature and bring to the boil. Reduce the heat and simmer.
- Drain the mushrooms. Put half in the liquidizer with a little wine and make a purée. Add to the contents of the casserole, together with the rest of the mushrooms.
- Stir and simmer for an hour. Adjust the seasoning. Allow to cool.
- Slowly reheat the coq-au-vin and serve.

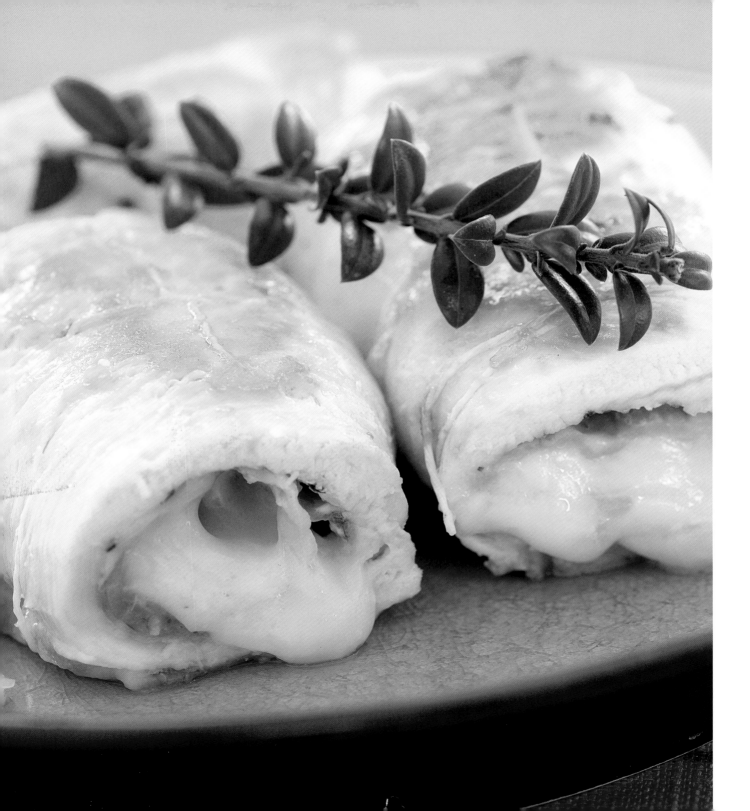

Lamb chops with mint

Serves 4

Preparation: 20 minutes
Cooking time: 10 minutes

- 8 lamb chops
- 1 tablespoon olive oil
- Herbes de Provence
- Salt, pepper
- A few leaves mint

- Brush the cutlets with olive oil and marinate for 15 to 20 minutes.
- Mix the herbes de Provence with some of the mint, finely chopped.
- Dip the cutlets in the herbs so they are completely coated. Season with salt and pepper.
- Cook under a hot grill and serve garnished with mint leaves.

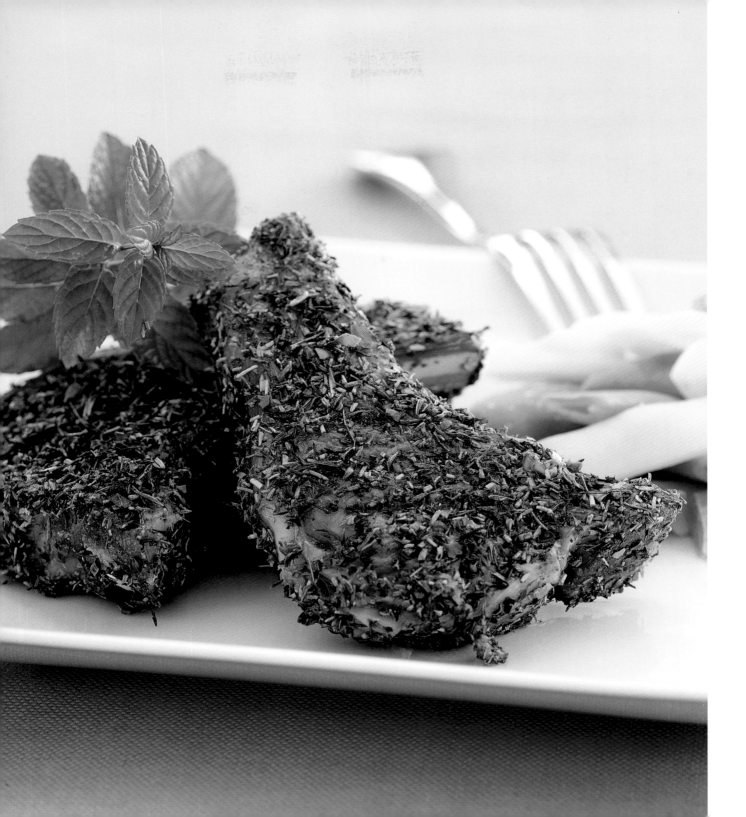

Pork chops with cream of mustard sauce

Serves 4

Preparation: 10 minutes
Cooking time: 20 minutes

- 4 large pork chops (or 8 small chops)
- 80 g (3oz) low fat crème fraîche or soya cream
- 3 tablespoons strong French mustard
- 1 tablespoon capers (preferably salted)
- 1 tablespoon goose fat
- Salt, pepper

- In a bowl, mix the crème fraîche, mustard and rinsed capers.
- Over a medium to high heat, melt the goose fat in a large frying pan and brown the chops for about 7 to 8 minutes on each side. Season with salt and pepper.
- Pour the sauce over the chops. Cover the pan and allow to simmer on a very low heat for about 10 minutes.
- Serve on warm plates.

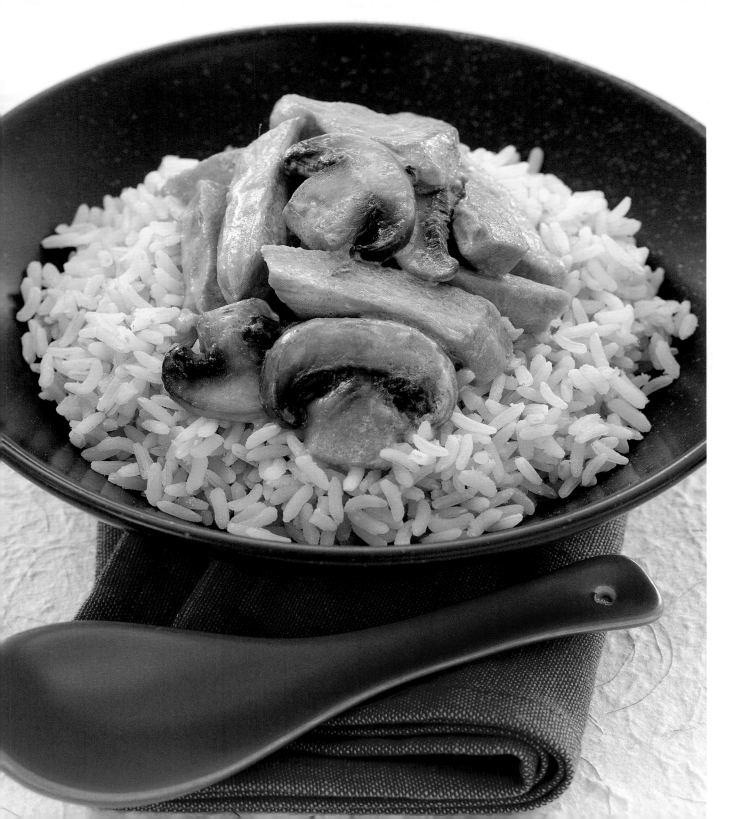

Entrecote steaks
Bordeaux style Serves 4

Preparation: 15 minutes
Cooking time: 30 minutes

- 2 entrecote steaks weighing 16oz and 2in thick (500 g and 4cm thick)
- 7fl oz (20 cl) red Bordeaux wine
- 4fl oz (10 cl) strong meat stock
- 4oz (100 g) tinned button mushrooms
- 5 shallots – chopped
- 4 tablespoons goose fat
- 1 sprig thyme
- 2 bay leaves
- 1 bunch of chopped parsley
- Salt and freshly ground pepper

- In a casserole heat 2 tablespoons of goose fat. Fry the shallots lightly for 2 to 3 minutes. Add a little red wine to moisten and then add the thyme, bay leaves, and stock. Season with salt and pepper. Over a strong heat with the lid removed, reduce the liquid by half.
- Drain the mushrooms, place in a liquidizer with a little olive oil, and reduce to a purée.
- Add this purée to the sauce in the casserole.
- In a large frying pan, heat the rest of the goose fat. Add the steaks and sear on both sides. Season with salt and pepper, and cook until the meat is either rare, medium or well done, according to individual taste.
- Deglaze the frying pan with a little red wine. Add the deglazing to the sauce.
- Cut the steaks into 4 or 8 slices and arrange on a warm serving dish. Cover with the bordelaise sauce and serve.

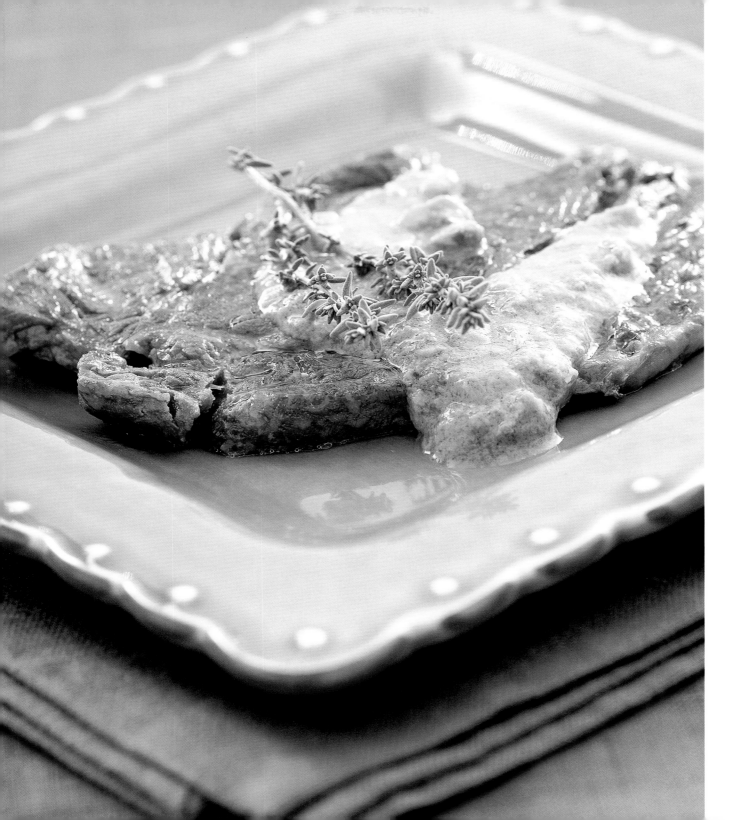

Shoulder of lamb cooked in lemon

Serves 6

Preparation: 15 minutes
Cooking time: 1 hour

- 2¼ lb (1 kg) boned shoulder of lamb
- 4 tablespoons olive oil
- 2 medium onions
- 1 clove garlic
- 2 tablespoons paprika
- 2 tablespoons chopped parsley
- 3 tablespoons lemon juice
- Lemon zest
- Salt, pepper

- Cut the lamb into 3 cm cubes and fry in a flameproof casserole, on a high heat in the olive oil. Once the meat is well browned, remove from the casserole and put on one side.
- In the same casserole, fry the finely chopped onions and garlic. Add the paprika, chopped parsley, lemon juice and zest of lemon and then replace the meat in the casserole.
- Season with salt and pepper, cover and simmer gently for 1 hour, adding a little water if necessary.
- Serve hot.

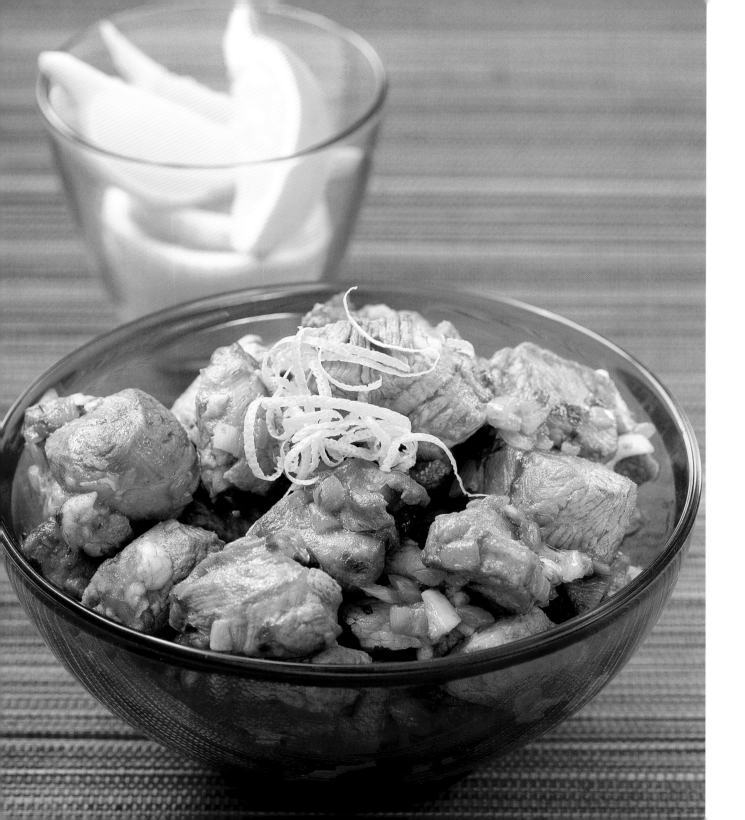

Veal escalope
with parma cream Serves 4

Preparation: 15 minutes
Cooking time: 35 minutes

- 4 escalopes weighing about 21oz (600 g)
- 6 slices Parma ham
- 1 onion
- 5fl oz (15 cl) low fat crème fraîche or soya cream
- 1 tablespoon olive oil
- Goose fat
- Salt, pepper, Cayenne Pepper

- In a non-stick frying pan, cook the slices of Parma ham over a low heat (1 to 2 minutes on each side), making sure they are in overall contact with the bottom of the pan.
- Dry them in the oven at 130°C (260°F, gas mark ½).until completely stiff and brittle. Cut into pieces and reduce to a powder in the blender. Reserve.
- Slice the onion finely and fry in a little olive oil over a low heat. Add the Parma ham powder and the crème fraîche. Season with salt, pepper and a pinch of Cayenne pepper.
- Salt and pepper the escallops. Melt the goose fat in a frying pan and gently fry the escallops.
- To serve, arrange on a dish or even better, serve on individual warmed plates and coat with the Parma Cream.

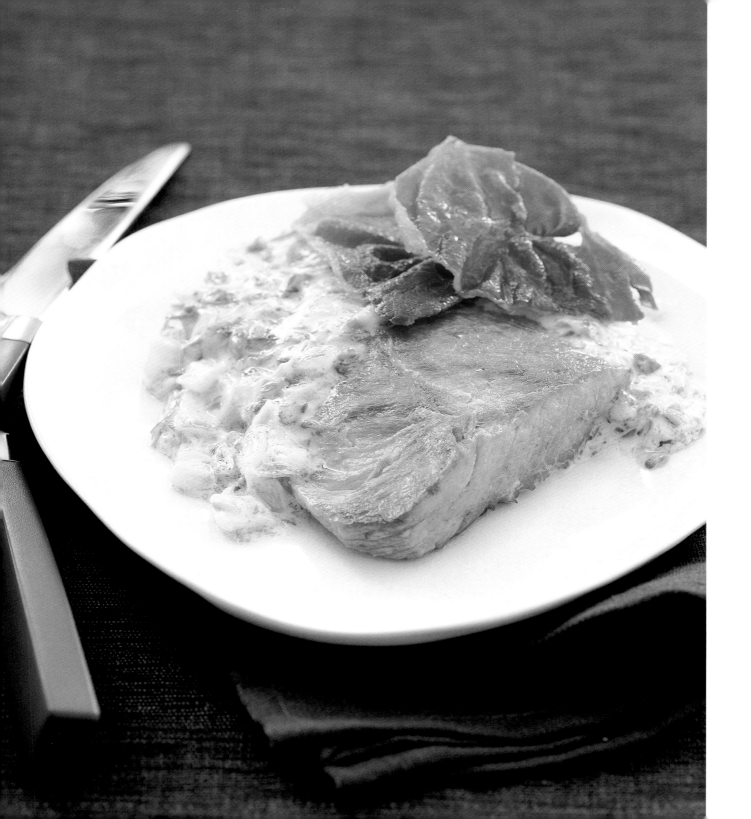

Turkey escalopes with cream

Serves 4

Preparation: 10 minutes
Cooking time: 20 minutes

- 4 good slices of turkey breast
- 4fl oz (10 cl) dry white wine
- 1 small yoghurt
- 1 tablespoon mustard
- Goose fat
- 1 tablespoon freshly chopped parsley
- Salt, pepper

- Fry the turkey slices in the goose fat over a medium heat till golden brown. Season with salt and pepper. Reserve and keep warm on the serving dish.
- Deglaze the pan with the white wine. Boil down slightly, then add the yoghurt mixed with the mustard. Stir over a gentle heat.
- Coat the escallops with the sauce and sprinkle with parsley.

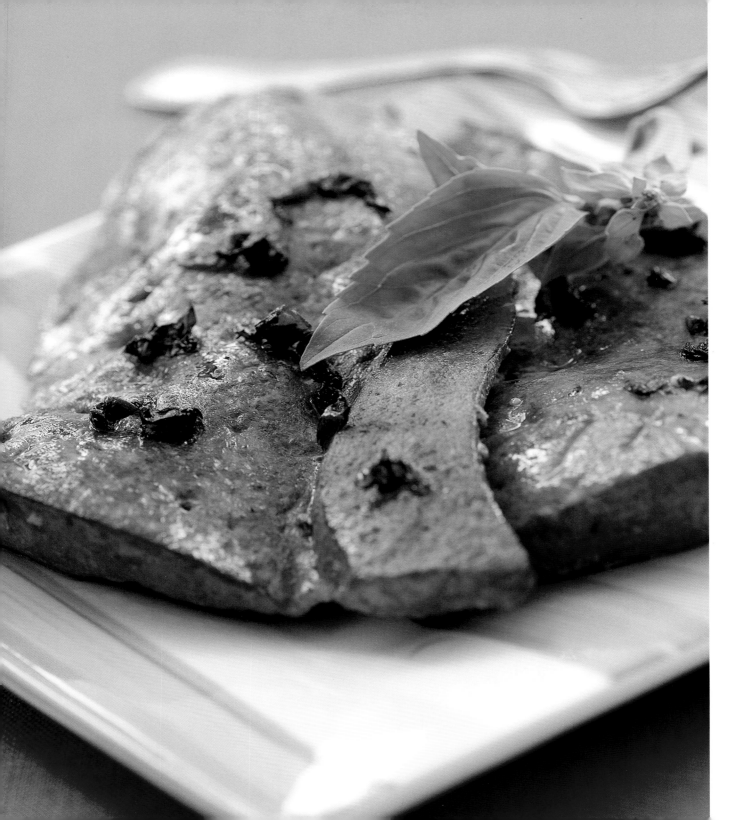

Calf's liver with onions

Serves 4

Preparation: 15 minutes
Cooking time: 15 minutes

- 4 slices calf's liver (6oz or 170 g each)
- 10 small onions
- Olive oil
- Goose fat
- 4fl oz (10 cl) low fat whipping cream or soya cream
- 1 tablespoon balsamic vinegar
- Salt, freshly ground pepper

- Slice the onions. Heat a small amount of olive oil in a large non-stick frying pan. Add the onions. Then season with salt and pepper. Do not brown the onions, but cook until almost transparent.
- In another frying pan, cook the slices of liver in the goose fat. Season with salt, pepper, reserve and keep warm.
- Deglaze the second frying pan with the balsamic vinegar and the cream. Add the cooked onions and stir well into the mixture.
- Serve on warm plates, coating the liver with the onion sauce.

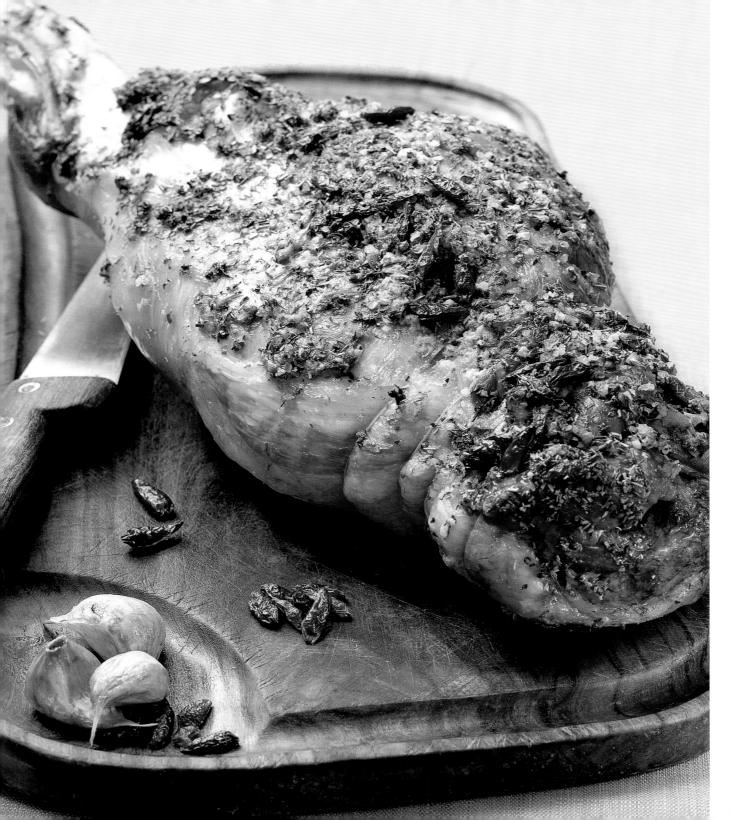

Rabbit with green olives

Serves 6

Preparation: 20 minutes
Cooking time: 1 hour

- 2 saddles of rabbit (800 g or 28oz each)
- 7oz (200 g) green olives
- 2 tablespoons tomato concentrate
- 3 cloves garlic
- 1 bouquet garni (thyme, rosemary, bay leaf)
- 2 onions
- 4oz (100 ml) olive oil
- 14oz (400 ml) white wine
- 2 sprigs fresh basil
- Salt, pepper

- Plunge the olives into unsalted boiling water for 1 to 2 minutes. Rinse in cold water, drain and remove the stones.
- Joint the rabbit.
- In a flameproof casserole, brown the pieces in olive oil on a high heat, then remove and replace with the sliced onions.
- When these are golden, drain on absorbent kitchen paper.
- Discard the cooking fat and pour in the white wine.
- Return the rabbit and onions to the casserole and add the tomato concentrate, half the olives, the peeled garlic cloves, and the bouquet garni. Season with salt and pepper.
- Cover and simmer for three quarters of an hour. Add the remainder of the olives 15 minutes from the end of the cooking time. Before serving, remove the bouquet garni and sprinkle with chopped basil leaves.

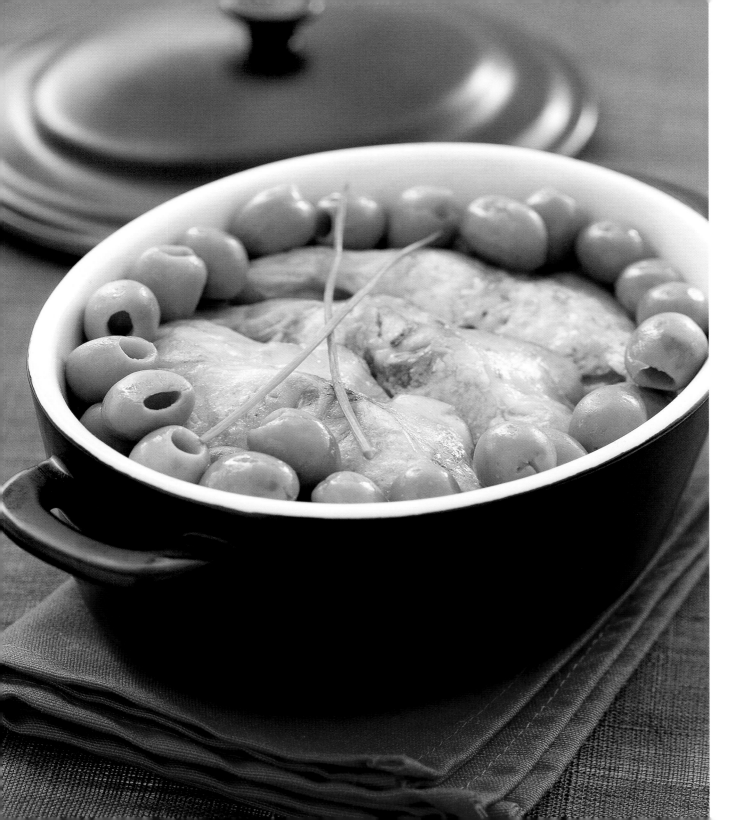

Rabbit with Mediterranean vegetables

Serves 6

Preparation: 20 minutes
Cooking time: 1 hour 20 minutes

- 1 rabbit (3¼ lb or 1.5 kg)
- 4 onions
- 4 aubergines
- 2 green peppers
- 2 red peppers
- 5 courgettes
- 6 tomatoes
- 7oz (200 ml) olive oil
- 1 bouquet garni
- 3 cloves garlic
- Salt, pepper

- Joint the rabbit and fry on high heat in 100 ml olive oil in a frying pan.
- Remove the rabbit pieces when they are browned and put on one side.
- Slice the onions and peppers and, in a flameproof casserole, fry on a high heat in the remainder of the olive oil. When they are golden, remove and replace with the aubergines and courgettes, sliced into rounds. Then return the onions and peppers to the casserole, followed by the rabbit joints.
- Plunge the tomatoes into boiling water for 30 seconds and skin. Remove the seeds and chop.
- Add to the casserole, along with the garlic, the bouquet garni and the salt and pepper.
- Cover and simmer gently for 1 hour.
- Remove the bouquet garni and serve.

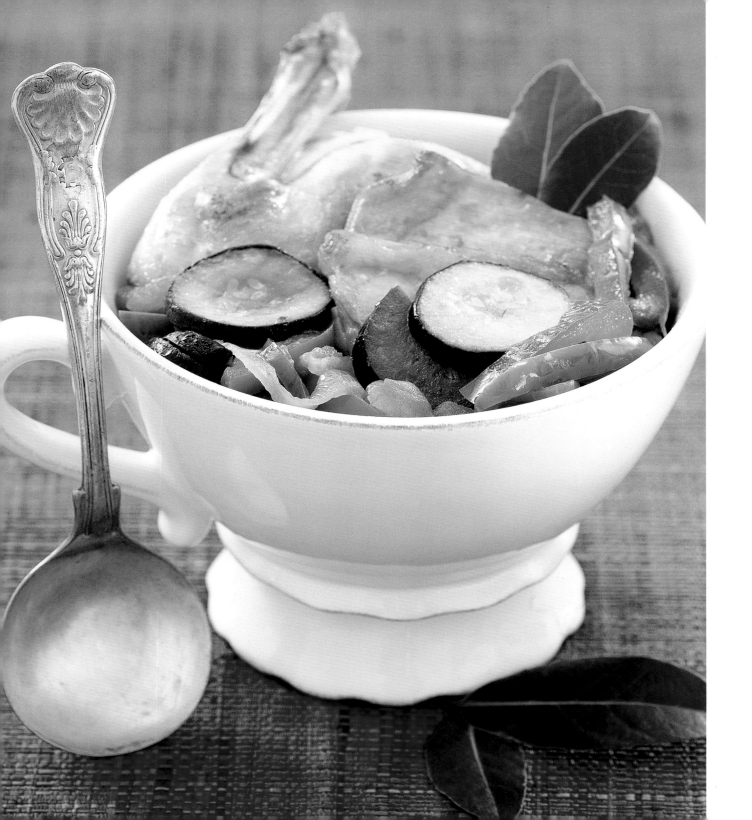

Duck breasts with olives

Serves 4

Preparation: 15 minutes
Cooking time: 20 minutes

- 1lb (500 g) green olives – stoned
- 3 duck breasts
- Salt, freshly ground pepper, Cayenne pepper
- Olive oil

- Purée 7oz (200 g) olives in the blender with 1 tablespoon of olive oil.
- Remove three-quarters of the fat covering the breasts.
- Use a third of the fat. Cut into cubes and melt slowly over a low heat. Discard the residue.
- Add the olive purée. Season with salt and pepper, then add the rest of the olives and cook for 5 minutes.
- For pink centres, fry the breasts in a non-stick pan for 6 minutes each side, starting with the fatty side. Vary the cooking time according to taste. Turn off the heat.
- Cut the breasts into slices 1cm (½in) thick, coat with the olive purée and serve on warm plates.

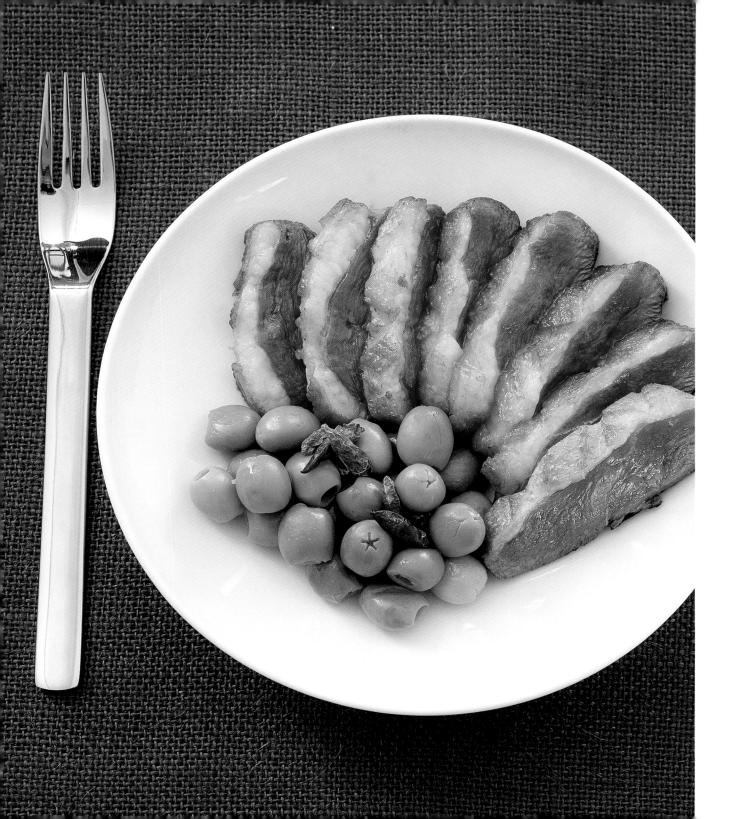

Duck breasts with orange

Serves 4

Preparation: 20 minutes
Cooking time: 15 minutes

- 3 duck breasts
- 3 oranges
- Juice of 2 oranges
- Zest of 1 orange
- Salt and freshly ground pepper

- Using a very sharp knife, remove the fat from the duck breasts, leaving a thin film on the meat which is barely visible.
- Dice the fat from one duck very finely. Discard the remainder.
- In a casserole, melt the diced fat over a low heat.
- Remove any residue with a slotted spoon.
- Peel the oranges and cut into slices. Fry gently for 3 minutes in the duck fat.
- In an ovenware dish, arrange the breasts fatty side uppermost. Season with salt.
- Spread the orange slices and zest around the duck, adding the juice of another 2 oranges.
- Place under a pre-heated grill (10cm – 4in) for 6 minutes.
- Transfer to a board and carve slices about 0.5cm (¼in) thick. Then, unless the breasts are preferred very pink, replace in the cooking dish and put in the oven at 100°C (200°F, gas mark ¼) for a further 2 or 3 minutes.
- Serve immediately in warm plates.

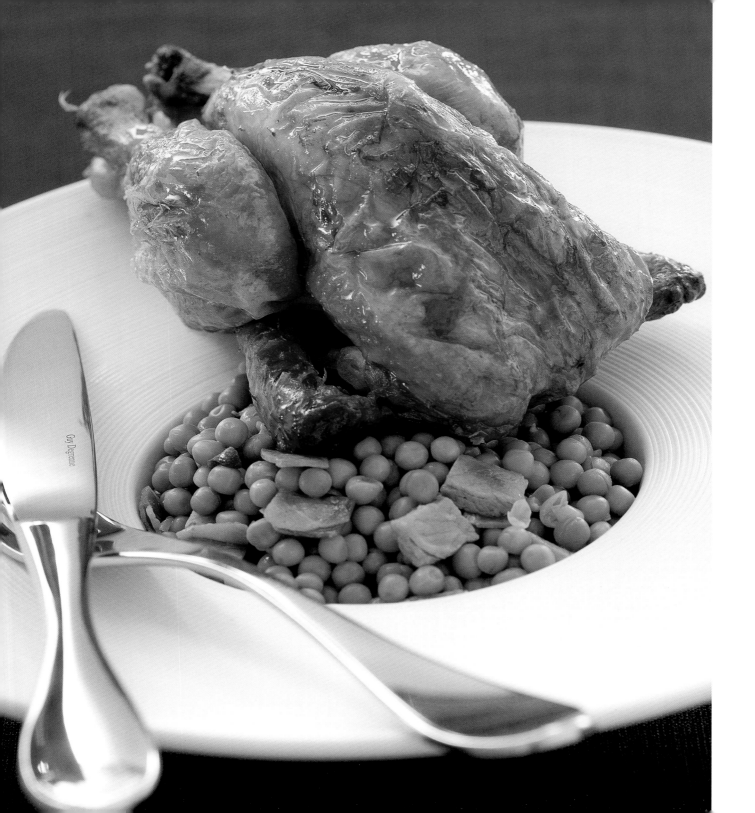

Traditional beef stew
Pot-au-feu

Serves 6

Preparation: 30 minutes
Cooking time: 3 hours

- 2¼ lb (1 kg) short rib with bone
- 21oz (600 g) shin of beef
- 2 bones (e.g. rib) without marrow
- 6 leeks
- 8 small turnips (navets)
- 2 heads celery
- 2 onions
- 2 cloves
- Salt, 10 peppercorns
- 1 bouquet garni

- Put the meat and bones in a large stockpot, cover with 4 litres of cold water, and add a table-spoon of salt. Bring to the boil and skim off the fat. Turn down the heat, cover and simmer for 1 hour.
- Then peel the onions and spike with the cloves. Add to the stockpot, along with the bouquet garni.
- One hour and a half into the cooking time, add the washed and prepared vegetables and 10 peppercorns. Add a little more water if necessary and simmer for a further hour and a half.
- Cut the meat up and serve surrounded by the vegetables.

Suggestion:
Allow the stock to cool, degrease it and remove the bouquet garni, and use as a soup.

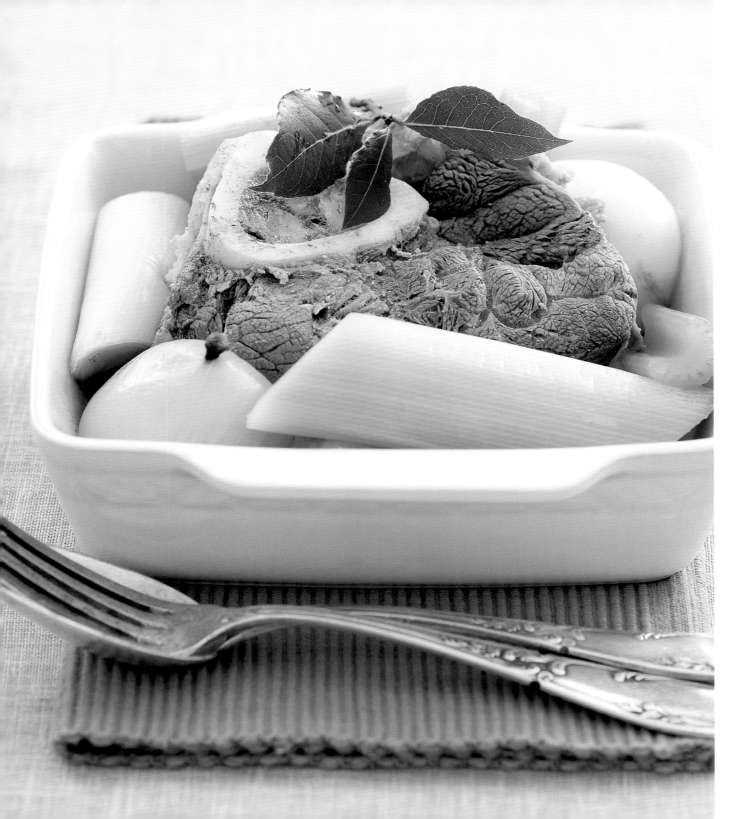

Chicken with garlic

Serves 4

Preparation: 20 minutes
Cooking time: 1 hour 20 minutes

- 1 free-range chicken weighing about 3lb (1.4kg), with liver
- 4 heads of garlic (about 20 cloves)
- 1 large celery stick
- Goose fat
- Salt, freshly ground pepper, Cayenne pepper

- Brown the liver gently in a pan with goose fat. Season with salt and pepper.
- Crush 5 cloves garlic and cut the celery stick into small pieces.
- Mix together in a blender liver, the crushed cloves of garlic, celery pieces, and 1 tablespoon of goose fat to make a purée. Season with salt and pepper.
- Stuff the chicken with the mixture.
- Place the chicken in an ovenware dish. Coat with the goose fat. Season with salt, pepper, and Cayenne pepper. Put in the oven at 210°C (420°F, gas mark 6½) and leave to cook for about 1 hour 15 minutes.
- After 20 minutes in the oven, baste the chicken with a glassful of hot salted water. Put the rest of the garlic which has not been peeled, around the chicken and leave to cook until the end.

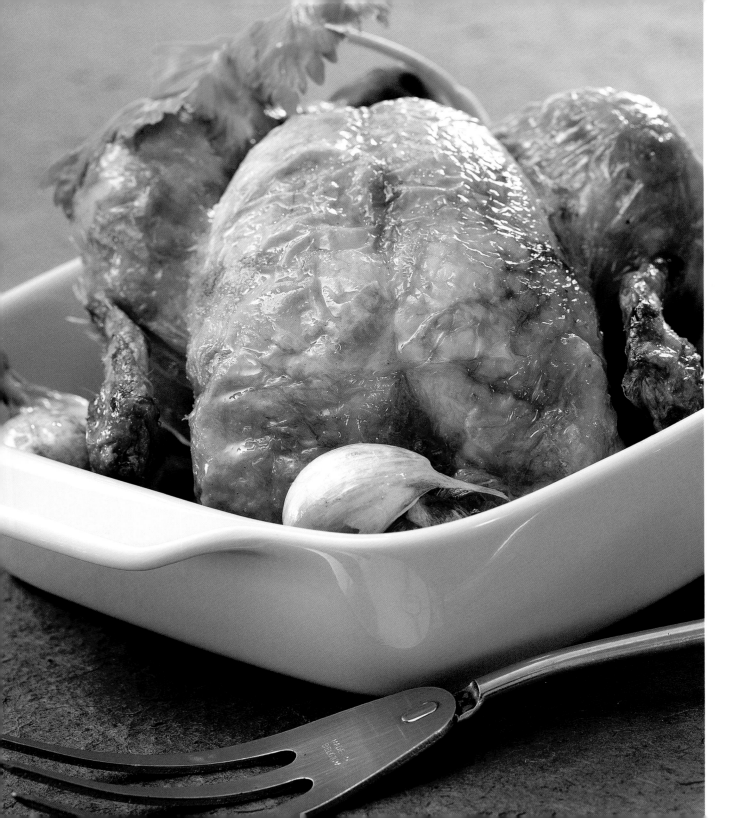

Chicken provençale

Serves 4 to 5

Preparation: 15 minutes
Cooking time: 40 minutes

- 1 free-range chicken weighing about 3lb (1.4kg)
- 1 large onion – sliced
- 4 cloves garlic – sliced
- 9fl oz (25 cl) chicken stock
- 3 tablespoons tomato purée
- Olive oil
- Salt, freshly ground pepper, Cayenne pepper, Herbes de Provence

- Cut the chicken into 8 pieces and arrange in an oven dish with the skin uppermost.
- Brush with olive oil. Season with salt, pepper, and Cayenne pepper.
- Cook under the grill for about 30 minutes. The skin should crisp slowly without getting charred, therefore care should be taken not to place it too close to the grill.
- In a casserole, brown the onions and the garlic in the olive oil. Pour over the stock and add the tomato purée. Stir well. Season with salt and pepper.
- Coat the pieces of chicken with the tomato sauce and sprinkle with some Herbes de Provence and put in the oven at 130°C (260°F, gas mark ½) for 5 or 10 minutes.
- Serve in the oven dish or in a warm serving dish.

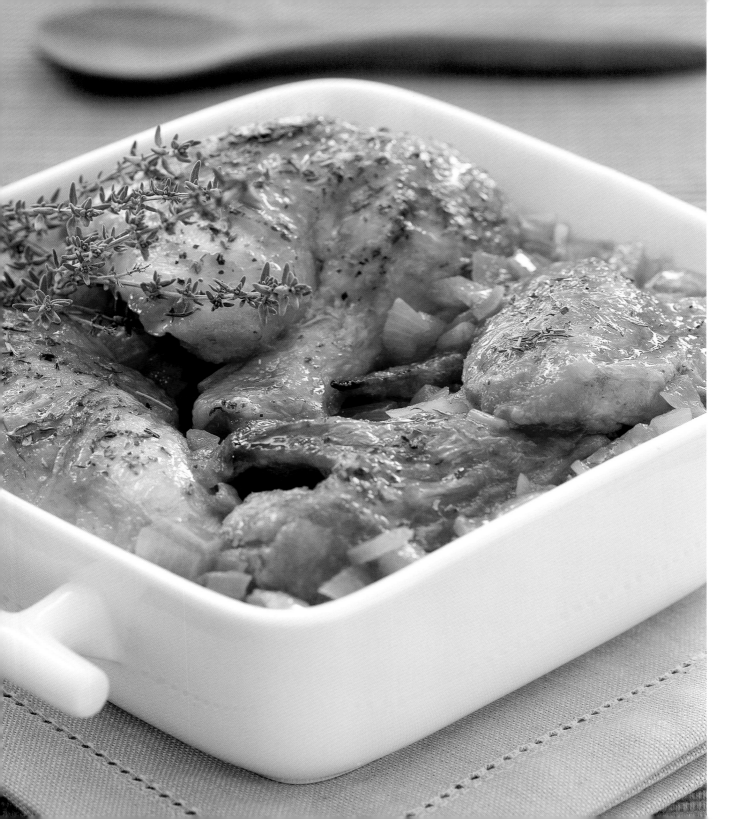

Chicken with apples and cider cream

Serves 4 to 5

Preparation: 20 minutes
Cooking time: 1 hour 40 minutes

- 1 free-range chicken weighing about 3¼ lb (1.5 kg)
- 2¼ lb (1 kg) apples
- 7fl oz (20 cl) dry cider
- 1 chicken stock cube
- 7fl oz (20 cl) low fat whipping cream or soya cream
- 2 teaspoons cinnamon
- Goose fat
- Salt, freshly ground pepper, Cayenne pepper

- Brush the chicken with a tablespoon of goose fat. Season with salt, pepper and Cayenne pepper and place in a pre-heated oven at 220°C (440°F, gas mark 7).
- Peel the apples and cut into pieces. Cook in the frying pan with goose fat, stirring regularly. Season liberally with salt, pepper, and cinnamon. Reserve.
- To make the Cream of Cider sauce, boil the cider in a pan and reduce by three quarters.
- Add the chicken stock cube and dissolve well. Then add the cream. Bring to the boil and turn off the heat. Correct the seasoning if necessary. In the last quarter of an hour, arrange the apples around the chicken.
- When ready, cut up the chicken, coat with the reheated cream of cider and serve with the cinnamon apples.

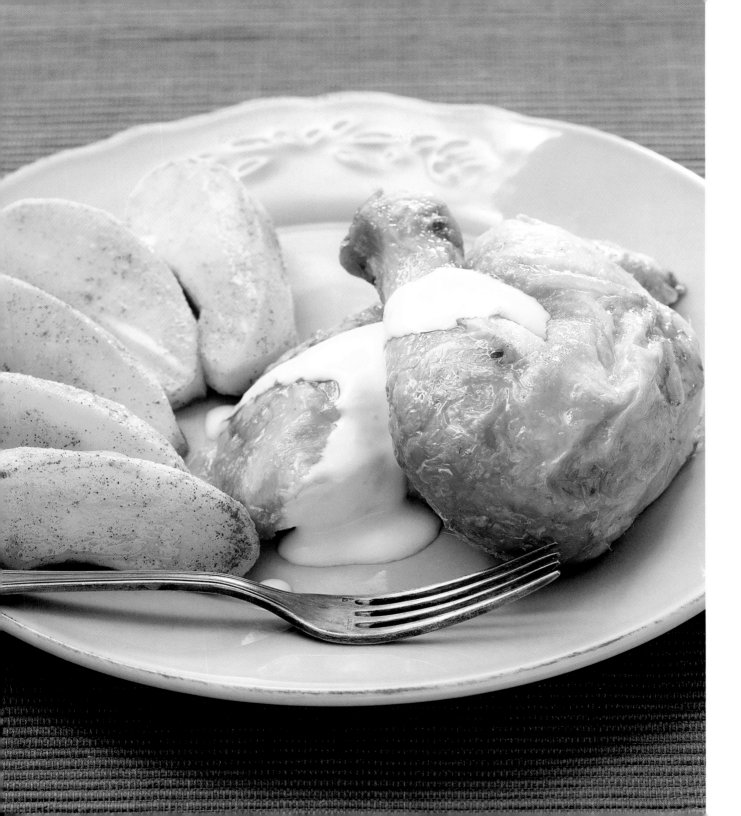

Chicken in a salt crust

Serves 4

Preparation: 10 minutes
Cooking time: 1 hour 40 minutes

- 1 free-range chicken weighing about 3¼ lb (1.5 kg)
- 5 to 6lb (2 - 3 kg) coarse salt

For the sauce:
- 10fl oz (30 cl) low fat whipping cream or soya cream
- 1 chicken stock cube

- In a cast iron stock-pot big enough to take the chicken with ease, lay a bed of salt 2cm (1in) thick. Lay the chicken on top and cover with salt, to a depth of 1.5cm (½ in).
- Place in a pre-heated oven at 180°C (360°F, gas mark 4) and cook for 1 hour 30 minutes.
- Crack the crust and take out the chicken when it will be ready to serve and eat.
- As there are no cooking juices, a sauce may be prepared by dissolving 1 cube of chicken stock in 10fl oz (30 cl) of whipping cream. To ensure the cube dissolves properly, grate it into a powder with the blade of a serrated knife. Avoid overheating the cream.

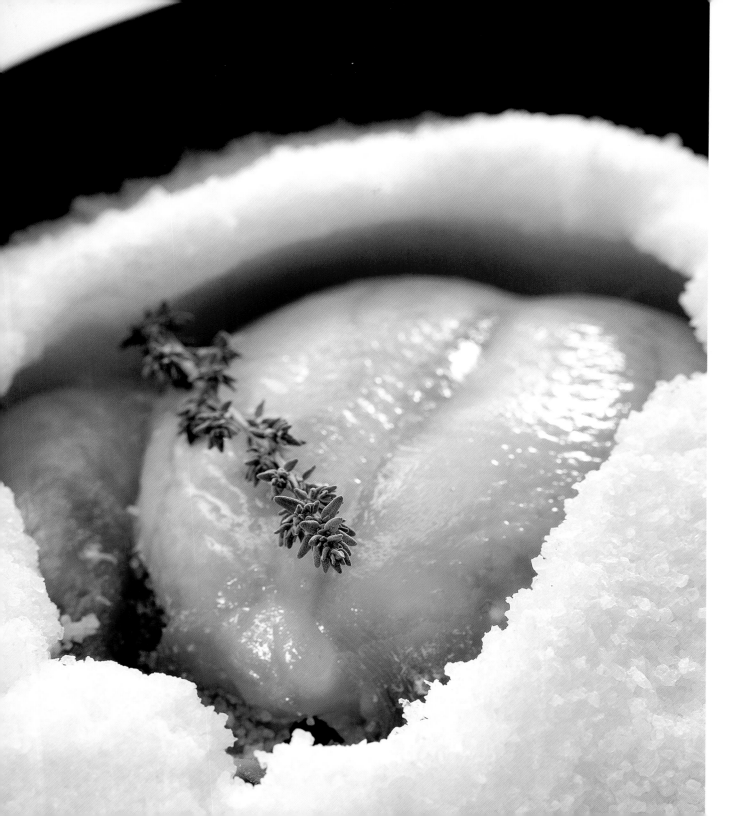

Roast duck breast

Serves 4

Preparation: 20 minutes
Cooking time: 25 minutes

- 3 duck breasts
- 2 cloves garlic
- Salt, pepper, Herbes de Provence

- Using a very sharp knife, remove the fat from one of the duck breasts.
- Season (salt, pepper, Herbes de Provence) each side and put togesther the roast. Put the duck breast without fat in the middle and arrange the breasts fatty side outwards.
- Secure the roast with a string.
- With a sharp pointed knife, make 4 deep cuts in the meat. Push the cloves of garlic (cut into two) deep into the flesh.
- Roast in the oven at 220°C (440°F, gas mark 7) for 25 minutes.
- After 10 minutes in the oven, discard the fat released and baste the duck with a glassful of hot salted water. Cut like a roast beef. The centre must be pink and warm.
- Serve with the cooking juice mixture with the cutting juice.

Suggestion:
Deglaze the tin with the low fat whipping cream (or soya cream) and season with salt, pepper and a pinch of Cayenne pepper.

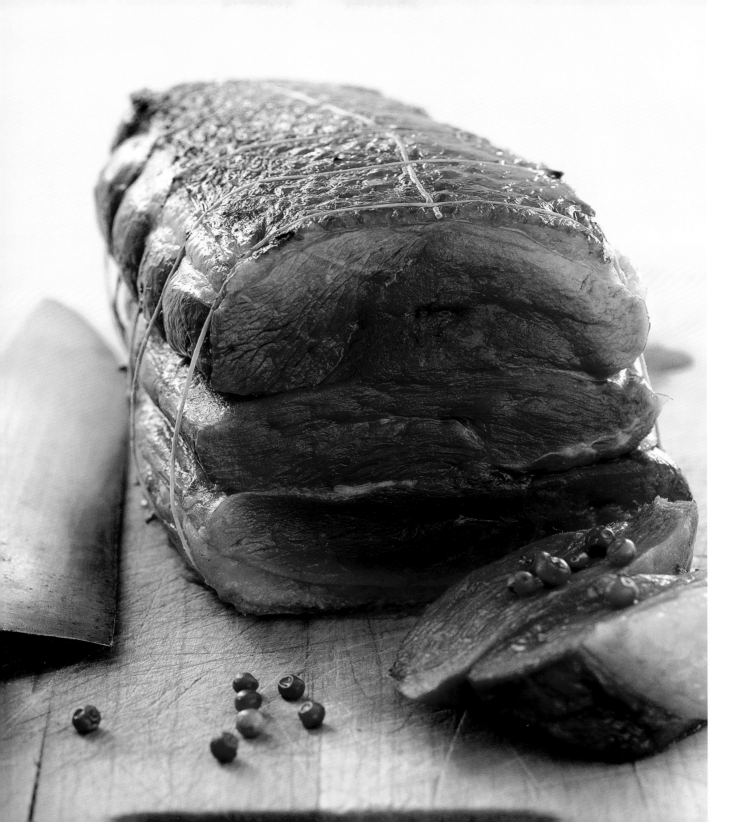

Roast pork with curry

Serves 4

Preparation: 15 minutes
Cooking time: 1 hour 15 minutes

- 4lb (1.8kg) pork fillet
- 4 cloves garlic – skinned
- 3 tablespoons goose fat
- 7fl oz (20 cl) low fat whipping cream or soya cream
- Curry
- Salt, freshly ground pepper

- With a sharp pointed knife, make 4 deep cuts in the meat. Push the cloves of garlic deep into the flesh.
- In a bowl, prepare a marinade with the melted goose fat. Season with salt, pepper and 1 tablespoon of curry. Mix well.
- Rub the mixture well into the meat.
- Place the meat in a tin and pour around the meat the rest of the marinade together with
- ½ glass of water. Roast in the oven at 220°C (440°F, gas mark 7) for 1 hour 15 minutes.
- Before serving, deglaze the tin with the whipping cream.

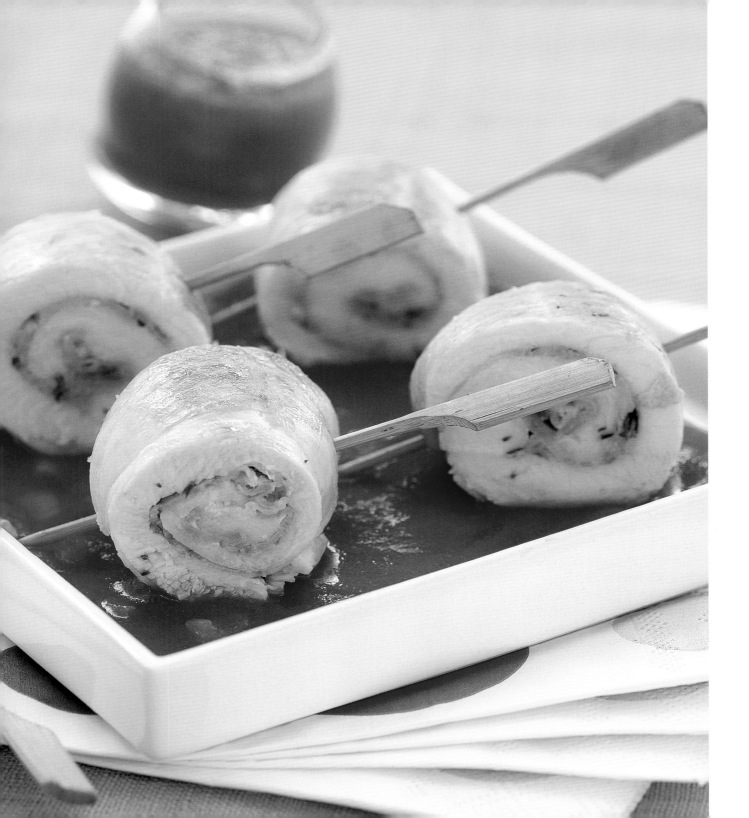

Tournedos provençale

Serves 4

Preparation: 15 minutes
Cooking time: 40 minutes

- 4 tournedos cut from the fillet, about 7oz (200 g) each
- 6 tomatoes
- 2 onions – sliced
- 3 red peppers
- 3 cloves garlic – finely sliced
- Olive oil, goose fat
- Salt, freshly ground pepper
- Herbes de Provence

- Cut the red peppers in half down their length. Remove the stalk and the seeds. Place under the grill skin-side up. When the skin has bubbled and is slightly charred, put them on one side to cool. Remove the skin and cut into strips about 1cm (½in) thick.
- Plunge the tomatoes into boiling water for about 30 seconds. Skin, deseed and cut into small cubes.
- In a large frying pan heat 2 or 3 tablespoons of olive oil over a low heat. Brown the onions stirring frequently. Add the garlic, diced tomatoes and strips of red pepper.
- Season with salt and pepper, and sprinkle a few Herbes de Provence sparingly over the top. Leave to cook over a gentle heat for 20 minutes.
- In another frying pan, melt a knob of goose fat and brown the tournedos 2 or 3 minutes each side. Season with salt and pepper.
- Pour the tomato sauce over the meat and continue cooking for 2 minutes.
- Serve hot.

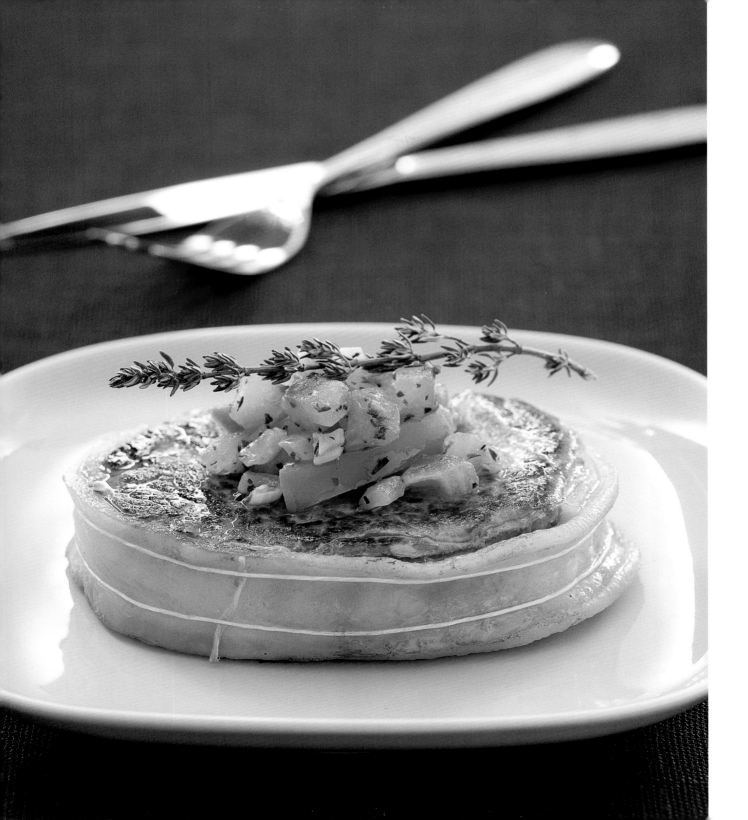

Tournedos with olives

Serves 4

Preparation: 15 minutes
Cooking time: 25 minutes

- 4 tournedos – 7oz (200 g) each
- 4 large tomatoes
- 20 stoned black olives
- 4 tablespoons anchovy paste
- Olive oil
- Salt, freshly ground pepper
- Herbes de Provence

- Cut each of the tomatoes into three. Place in an ovenware dish and brush with oil on both sides. Season with salt, pepper, and sprinkle with Herbes de Provence.
- Put under the grill until they are slightly browned. Reserve and keep warm.
- In a frying pan, fry the black olives in the olive oil.
- Brush the tournedos with the anchovy paste. Heat some olive oil in a frying pan and cook the meat for 2 or 3 minutes on each side. Do not salt.
- Serve the tournedos very hot with the tomatoes, olives and their cooking juices.

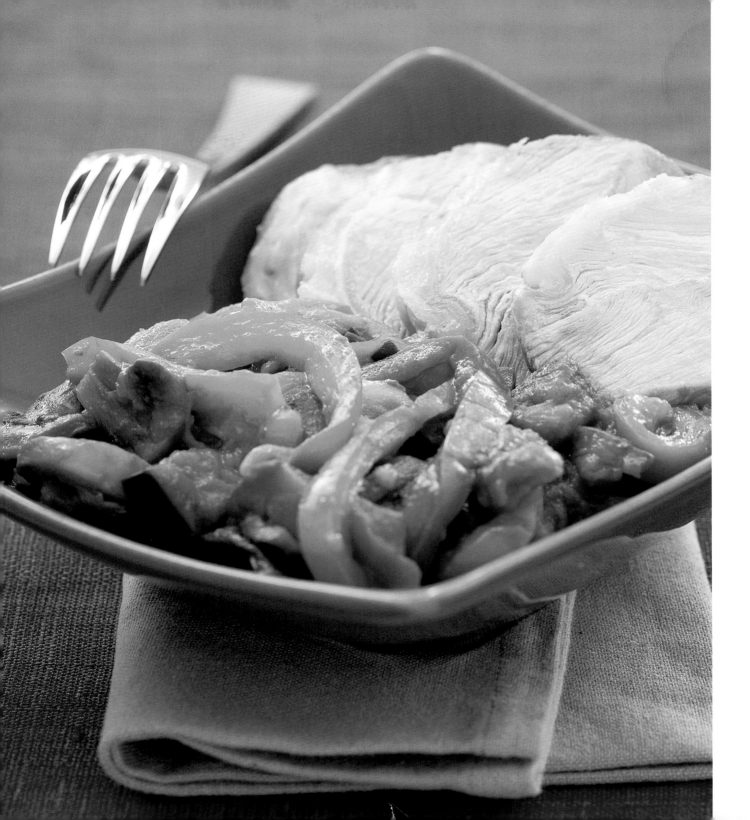

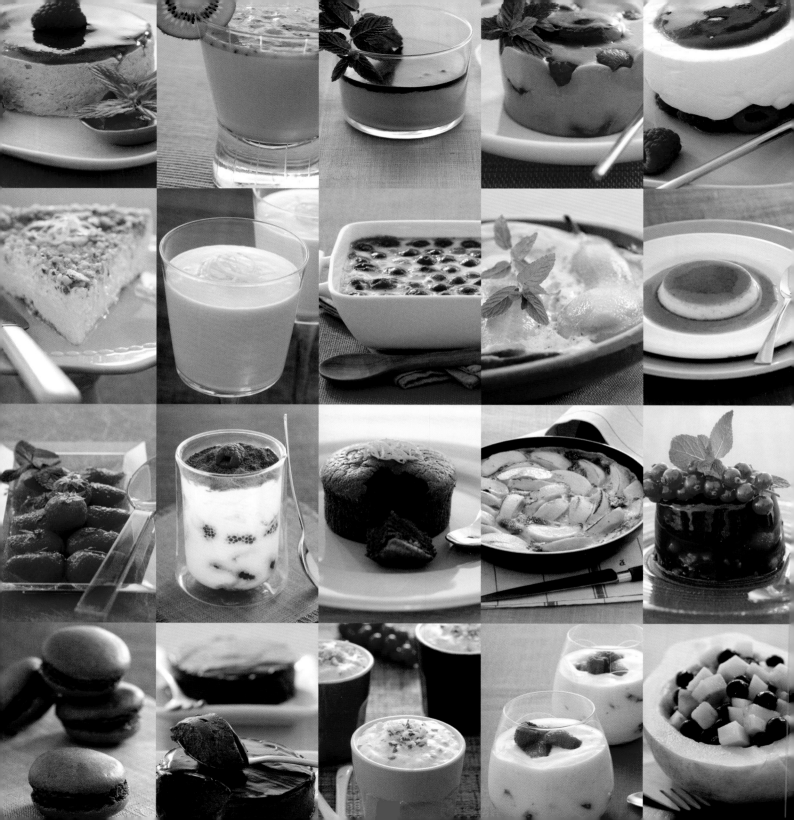

Desserts recipes

Apricot bavarois
with its coulis Serves 4

Preparation: 20 minutes
Cooking time: 15 minutes

- 26oz (750 g) apricots
- 5 leaves of gelatine – or the equivalent of agar-agar
- 9fl oz (25 cl) full milk
- 4oz (100 g) fructose
- 7fl oz (20 cl) whipping cream
- 2fl oz (5 cl) cognac

- Cut the apricots in half and remove the stones. Place in a steamer with the skin side facing downwards and cook for 10 minutes. Reserve and allow to cool.
- Bring the milk to the boil and then allow to cool for 10 minutes.
- Immerse the leaves of gelatine in cold water. Squeeze dry and then add to the milk.
Stir well and allow to stand for 15 minutes.
- Mix 50 g (2oz) of fructose with the cream and beat until stiff.
- Fold the whipped cream into the milk (which is just beginning to set) and add the cognac.
Stir gently with the whisk to obtain a smooth mixture.
- Take half the apricots, dice and fold into the mixture.
- Pour into ramekins or into rings 8 cm (3in) in diameter, and place in the fridge for 6 hours and allow to set.
- To make the coulis, combine the remaining apricots and fructose in a food processor.
Reserve and keep cool.
- Unmould onto individual plates and surround with the coulis.

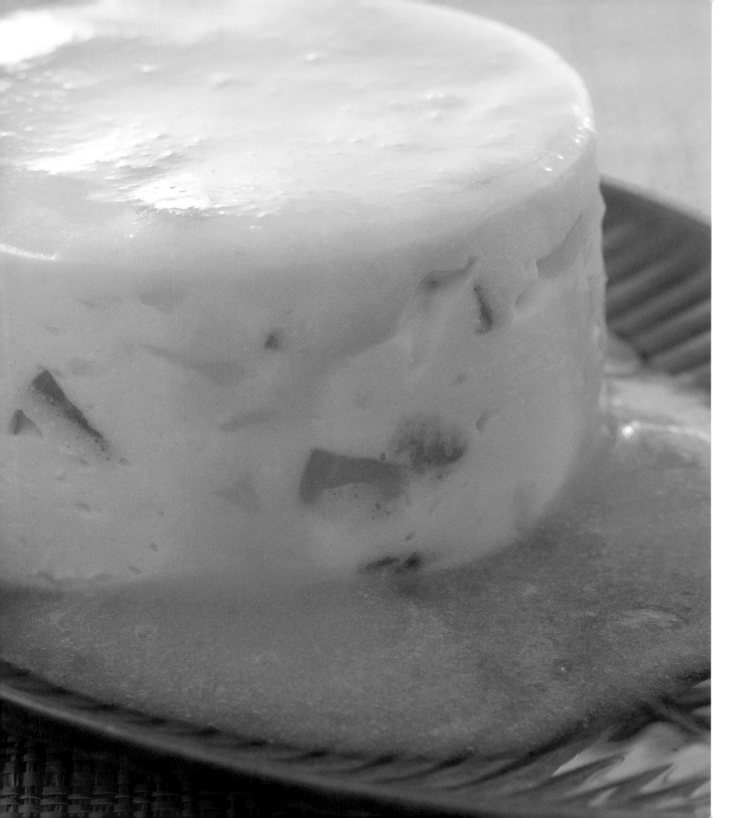

Raspberry bavarois

Serves 4

Preparation: 15 minutes
Refrigeration: 12 hours

- 1lb (500 g) raspberries
- 1 pint (1/2 litre) milk
- 4 egg yolks
- 3 tablespoons fructose
- 3 leaves of gelatine

- Bring the milk to the boil.
- Beat the egg yolks and fructose together in a large bowl.
- Gradually pour the milk into the bowl, stirring vigorously all the time. Return to a low heat and cook until the mixture thickens stirring continuously. Stir in the gelatine; first soften in cold water and drain.
- Blend 200 g (7oz) of the raspberries to a purée and combine this with the custard. Add 50 g (2oz) whole raspberries.
- Pour the mixture into ramekins or a charlotte mould and place in the refrigerator for 12 hours to set.
- Make a raspberry coulis with the remainder of the fruit. Turn out and coat with the coulis.

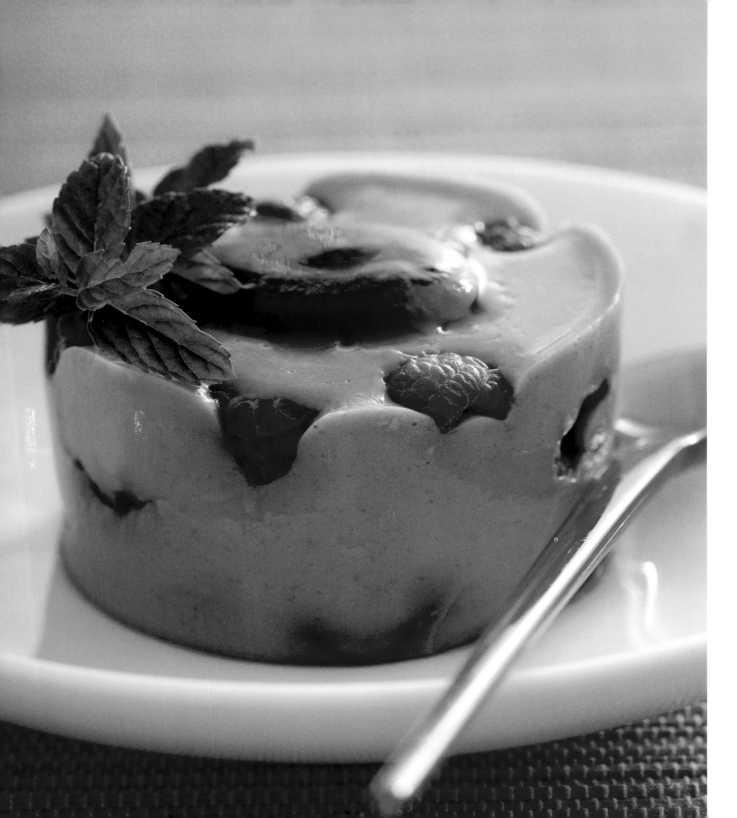

Raspberry bavarois with its coulis Serves 4

Preparation: 20 minutes
Cooking time: 15 minutes
Refrigeration: 6 hours

- 26oz (750 g) raspberries
- 1 lemon
- 3 tablespoons fructose
- 5oz (150 g) fromage frais
- 5fl oz (15 cl) low fat whipping cream
- 5 leaves of gelatine (or the equivalent of agar-agar)

- Liquidize the raspberries and put through a conical sieve to remove the pips if necessary.
- Add the lemon juice and fructose.
- Reserve a third of the mixture in the fridge, for making the coulis later.
- Drain the fromage frais.
- Soak the gelatine leaves in a bowl of cold water. Add to the two thirds of the raspberry purée. Mix with the fromage frais and the whipping cream.
- Pour into small moulds and place in the fridge for 6 hours or until the mixture begins to set.
- Turn out the moulds onto individual plates and surround the bavarois with the remaining coulis. Decorate eventually with a mint leaf and serve.

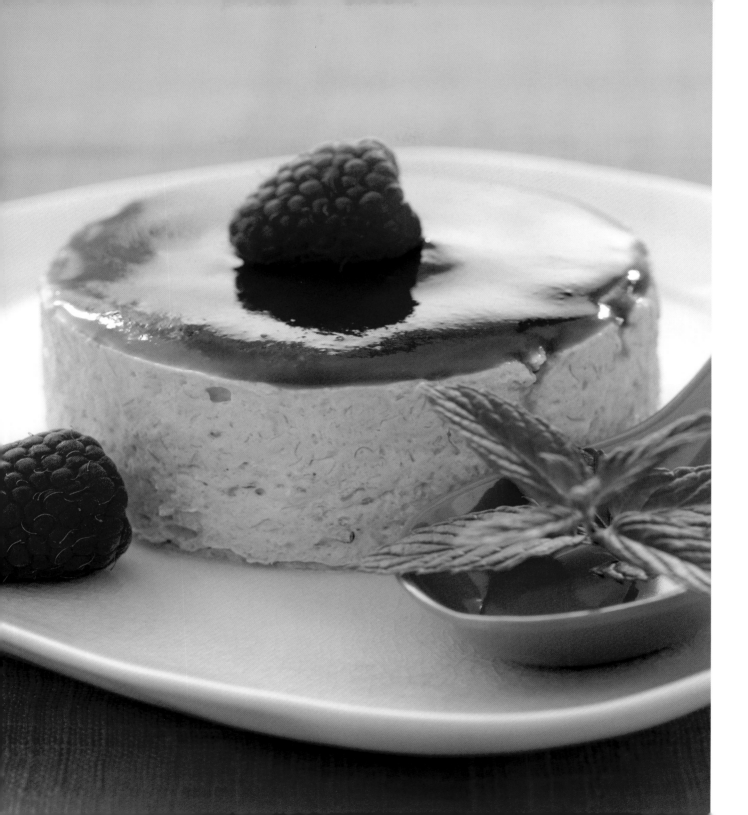

Mango bavarois
with a kiwi coulis Serves 6

Preparation: 15 minutes
Refrigeration: 12 hours

- 5 egg yolks
- 11oz (300 ml) full milk
- 11oz (300 g) peeled mango
- 3 leaves of gelatine
- 3 tablespoons fructose

For the kiwi coulis:
- 4 kiwis
- Juice of 1 lemon
- 2 tablespoons fructose

- Make an egg custard, as follows:
- Heat the milk, beat the eggs with the fructose in a large bowl, and gradually pour the milk into the bowl, whisking all the time. Return to a low heat, stirring continuously until the mixture thickens.
Stir in the gelatine; leaves must be previously softened in cold water and drained.
- Blend the mango to a smooth purée and stir it into the custard.
- Pour the mixture into a mould and leave in the refrigerator to set for 12 hours.
- Make a coulis by blending the kiwis with the lemon juice and fructose.
- Turn out the bavarois and serve with the kiwi coulis poured over.
.

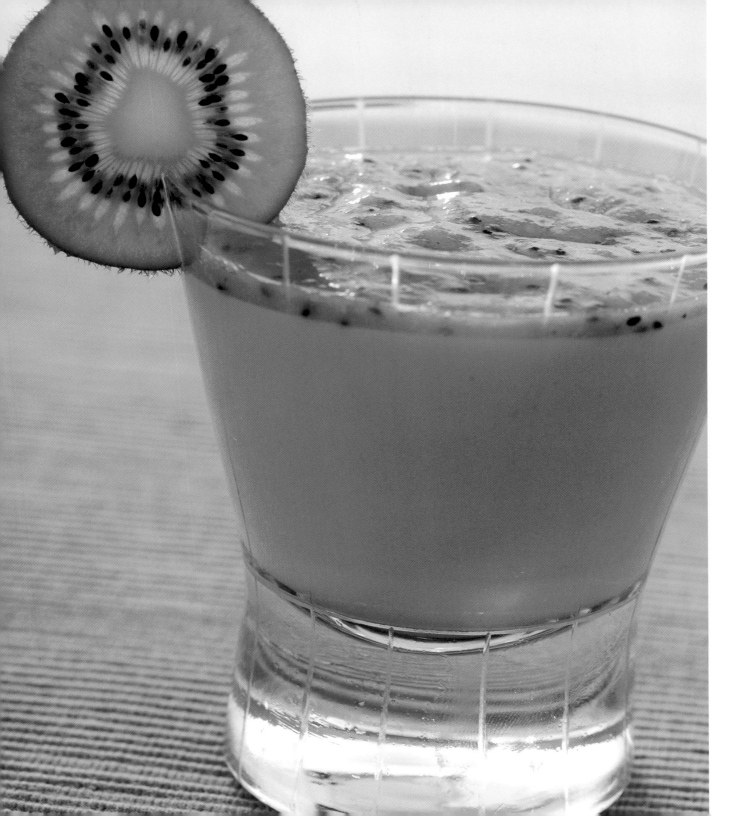

Vanilla and chocolate bavarois

Serves 6

Preparation: 15 minutes
Refrigeration: 12 hours

- 1¾ lb (750 ml) full cream milk
- 10 egg yolks
- 5 tablespoons fructose
- 1 vanilla pod
- 3 leaves of gelatine
- 2 teaspoons instant coffee
- 1 tablespoon rum
- 5oz (150 g) dark chocolate with 70 % minimum cocoa solids

- Boil the milk with the vanilla pod (sliced in half lengthways) for 10 minutes.
- Dilute the coffee in a few drops of the hot milk. Stir this into the rest of the milk, together with the rum.
- Beat the egg yolks with the fructose in a large bowl. Pour the milk into the bowl, stirring continuously. Return to a low heat and stir until the mixture thickens.
- Stir in the gelatine; leaves must be previously softened in cold water and drained. Pour the mixture into a mould and set in the refrigerator for 12 hours.
- Just before serving, melt the chocolate in a bain-marie, adding a little water. Allow to cool a little.
- Turn out the bavarois and serve with the lukewarm chocolate poured over.

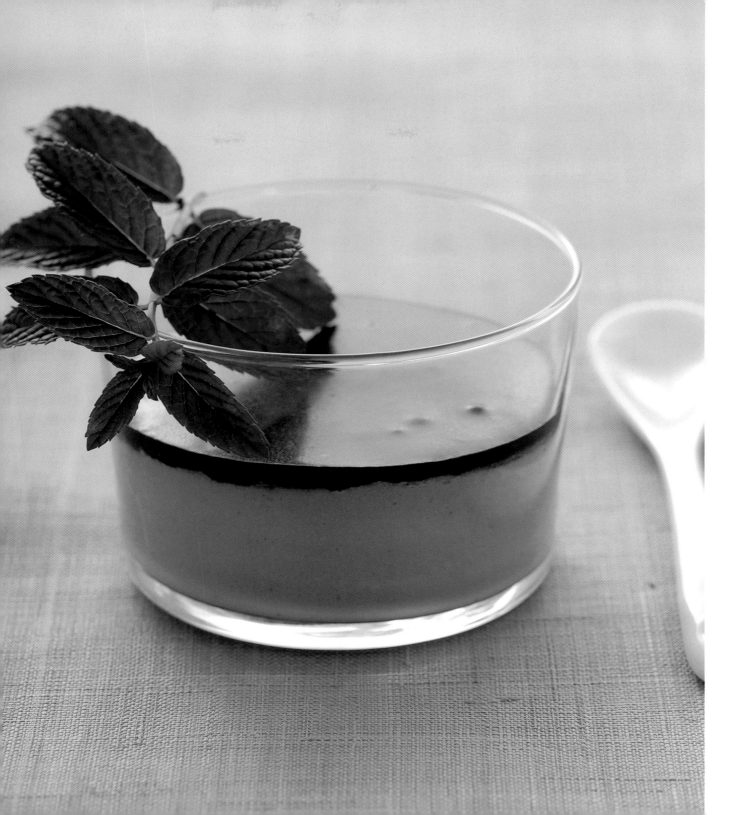

Blanc-Mangé with raspberry coulis Serves 5

Preparation: 20 minutes
Cooking time: 5 minutes

- 9oz (250 g) raspberries
- 14oz (400 g) fromage frais – strained
- 10fl oz (30 cl) whipping cream
- 4 tablespoons of sugar-free raspberry jam
- 6 leaves of gelatine (or the equivalent of agar-agar)
- 1 tablespoon fructose
- 1 tablespoon rum

- Whip the cream until stiff.
- Soften the gelatine leaves in rum which should be lukewarm.
- Mix well together the whipped cream, strained fromage frais, rum gelatine and raspberry jam.
- Arrange some raspberries at the bottom of each mould and pour the rum mixture over the top and place in the fridge to set.
- Prepare the coulis by liquidizing the remaining raspberries with the fructose. Strain through a sieve.
- To serve, unmold the bavarois onto individual plates and coat with the coulis.

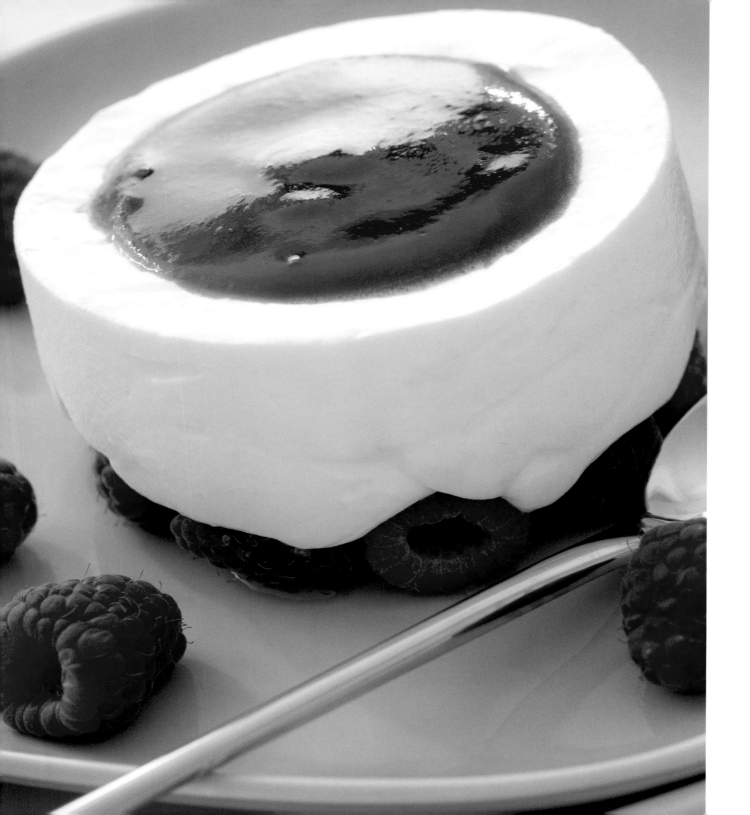

Apple scramble
with cinnamon Serves 4

Preparation: 30 minutes
Cooking time: 35 minutes

- 8 nice apples
- 3 whole eggs + 3 yolks
- 4 tablespoons fructose
- 2fl oz (5 cl) calvados
- 5fl oz (15 cl) low-fat crème fraîche
- Cinnamon powder

- Peel the apples. Quarter and remove the core.
- Cook in the steamer for about 20 minutes. Drain well.
- In a large bowl, beat the egg, yolks, and fructose.
- Add the apples, calvados and crème fraîche. Sprinkle with cinnamon. Continue to beat with a whisk until the mixture has a uniform consistency.
- Pour into a large non-stick pan and cook over a very, very low heat – as for making scrambled eggs stirring continuously with a spatula. Take the pan off the heat and pour the mixture which should still be slightly moist, into low ovenware dishes or ramekins.
- Sprinkle cinnamon over the top and when quite cool, place in the fridge for 2 or 3 hours.

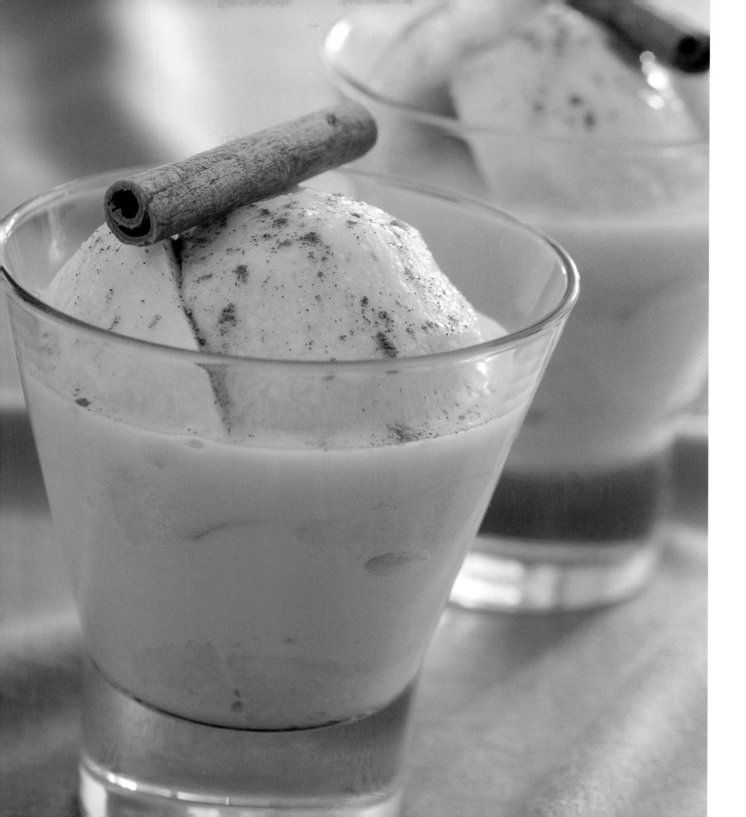

Chestnut and chocolate mousse

Serves 5

Preparation: 20 minutes
Cooking time: 15 minutes

- 3¼ lb (1.5 kg) chestnuts
- 7oz (200 g) chocolate with 70% cocoa solids
- 4oz (100 g) low fat crème fraîche
- 3 tablespoons fructose
- 18fl oz (50 cl) milk
- 1 vanilla pod (or 2cc of essence)
- 3fl oz (7 cl) cognac

- Peel the chestnuts.
- Boil for 5 minutes to ease removal of the inner skin.
- Then cook over a low heat in the vanilla milk for about 30 minutes, until soft.
- Drain and reduce to a purée using the potato masher.
- Melt the chocolate with the cognac in a bain-marie.
- In a large bowl, mix the chestnuts, melted chocolate, crème fraîche and fructose together thoroughly.
- Line a mould with aluminium foil which has been lightly greased.
- Pour in the mixture. Cover with plastic film and put in the fridge for at least 5 hours.
- Turn out and serve onto a melted chocolate base coating individual plates. Eventually, decorate also with whipped cream.

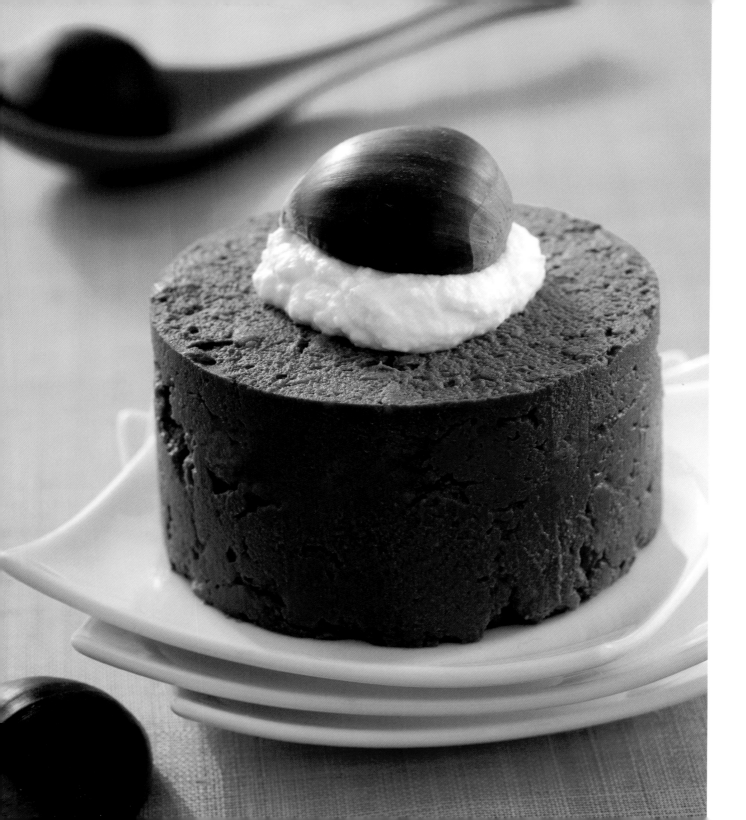

Cheese Cake with ginger Serves 4

Preparation: 20 minutes
Cooking time: 50 minutes

- 2¼ lb (1 kg) cream cheese (Philadelphia)
- 2 eggs + 1 egg yolk
- 5oz (150 g) fructose
- Juice of 1 lemon
- 2 teaspoons ginger spice
- 4oz (100 g) almonds very coarsely chopped
- Olive oil

- Preheat the oven to 125°C (250°F, gas mark ½).
- Put the cream cheese in a bowl.
- Add the fructose, the eggs, and the ginger.
- Liquidize the mixture or whip vigorously.
- Add the lemon juice and continue beating for 3 minutes.
- Oil a 22/23 cm mould with detachable bottom.
- Sprinkle the inside of the mould with 50 g (2oz) powder almonds.
- Pour in the mixture and sprinkle with the rest of almonds.
- Put in the oven and cook for 50 minutes.
- Allow to cool to room temperature and then refrigerate for 3 to 4 hours.
- Serve lukewarm or cold.

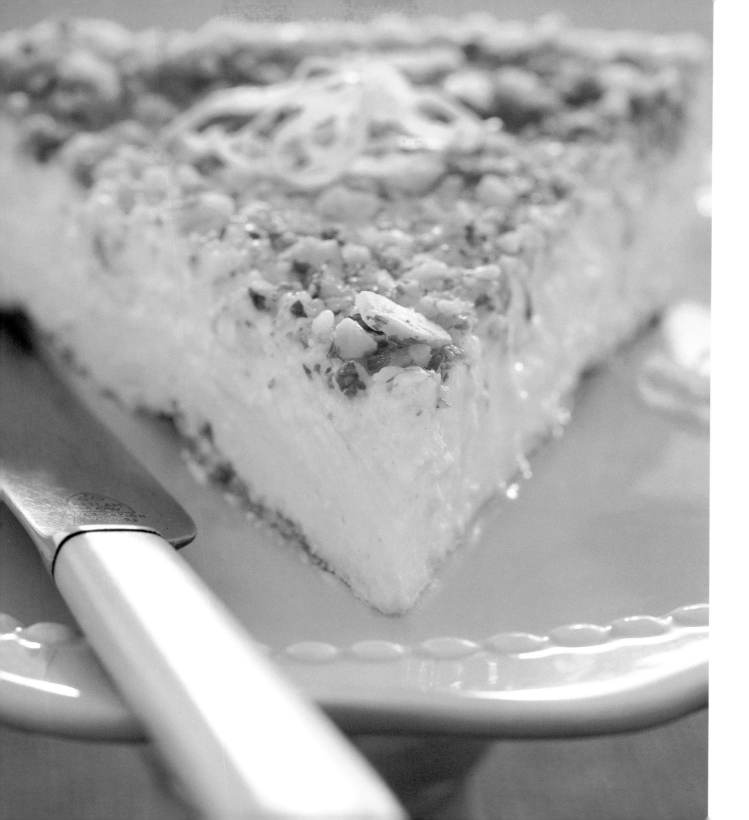

Lemon mousse

Serves 4

Preparation: 20 minutes
Cooking time: 20 minutes

- 3 lemons
- 5 egg yolks + 1 whole egg
- 7fl oz (20 cl) full milk
- 7fl oz (20 cl) whipping cream
- 5oz (150 g) fructose
- 3 leaves of gelatine (or equivalent of agar-agar)

- Grate the lemon zest.
- Beat the eggs with the fructose, juice of 3 lemons and the zest.
- Heat the milk and allow to cool for a few minutes.
- Gently pour the milk on the egg and lemon mixture, beating vigorously with a whisk.
- Return to a very low heat (preferably a bain-marie) and allow the mixture to thicken while stirring constantly with the whisk. Allow to cool for 10 minutes.
- Soak the leaves of gelatine in cold water for a few minutes. Squeeze dry and add to the mixture, stirring in well with the whisk. Allow to cool for 30 minutes.
- Whip the cream and fold into the mixture.
- Pour into ramekins. Cover with plastic film and refrigerate for 5 to 6 hours before serving.

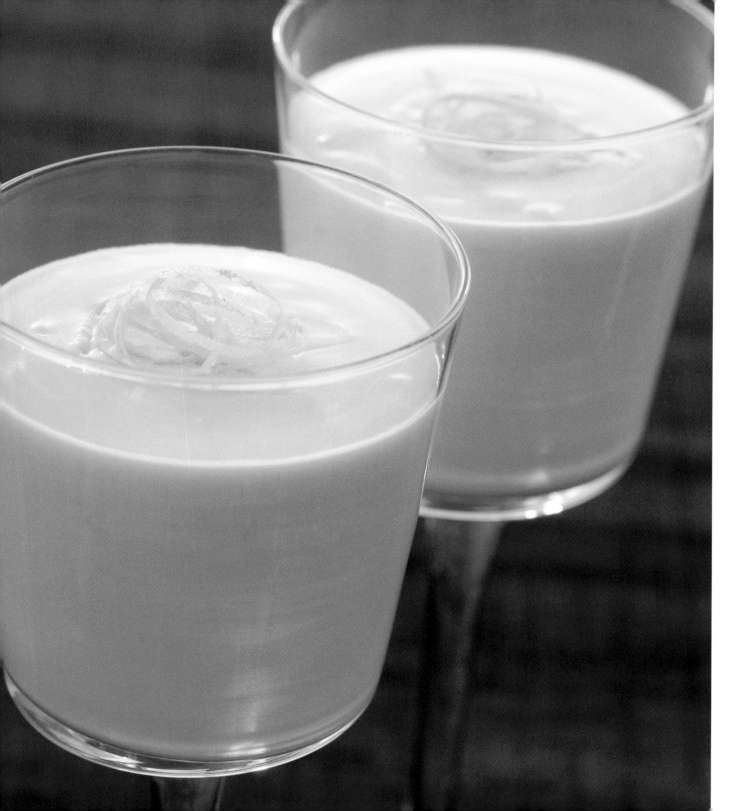

Cherry flan

Serves 5

Preparation: 15 minutes
Cooking time: 60 minutes

- 26oz (750 g) stoned cherries
- 7fl oz (20 cl) milk
- 7fl oz (20 cl) low fat whipping cream
- 2oz (60 g) fructose
- 6 eggs
- 6 tablespoons rum
- Vanilla extract

- Heat the milk and the whipping cream without boiling. Allow to cool.
- In a large bowl, beat together the eggs with the fructose. Pour in the milk, stirring constantly.
- Add a few drops of vanilla extract and the rum.
- Arrange the cherries in a 28 cm (11in) flan dish. Pour the mixture over the cherries.
- Cook for 50 minutes in the oven at 130°C (260°F, gas mark ½). Allow to cool before putting in the fridge. Chill completely before serving.

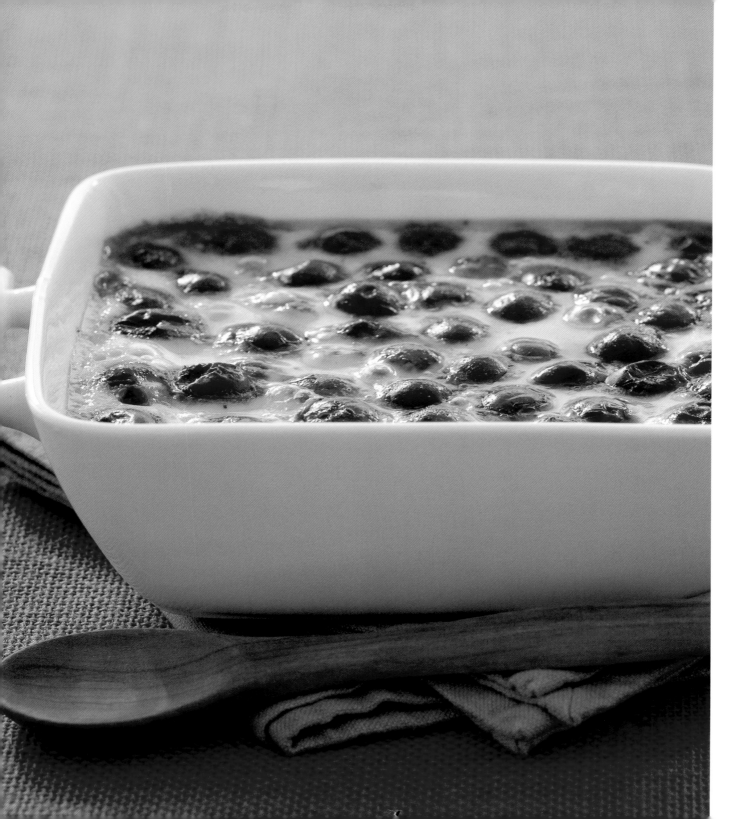

Pear flan

Serves 4

Preparation: 20 minutes
Cooking time: 45 minutes

- 5 good-size pears
- 1 vanilla pod (vanilla seeds)
- 3oz (80 g) fructose
- 3 eggs + 1 egg yolk
- 9fl oz (25 cl) milk
- 5fl oz (15 cl) low fat crème fraîche
- 1fl oz (2 cl) pear brandy or rum
- Oil

- Preheat the oven to 200°C (400°F, gas mark 6).
- Peel the pears, quarter and remove the cores. Slice each quarter into two.
- Oil a flan dish.
- In a large bowl, beat together the eggs with the fructose and the vanilla seeds.
- Add the milk and the pear brandy to the crème fraîche and fold into the eggs.
- Arrange the pears in the flan dish. Pour the mixture over the pears.
- Put in the oven and cook for 40 to 45 minutes.

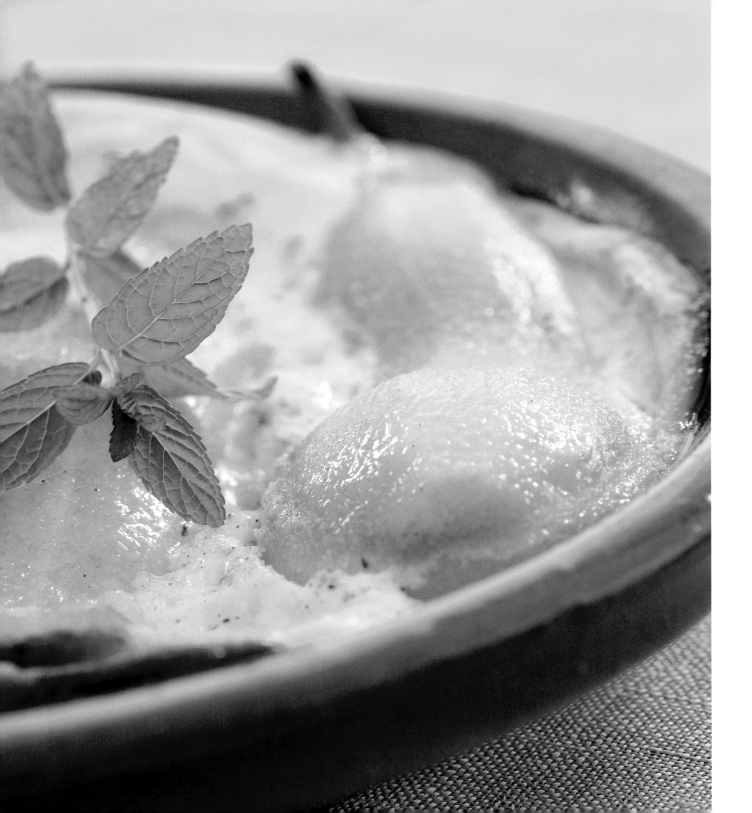

Cream caramel
with fructose
Serves 6

Preparation: 15 minutes
Cooking time: 55 minutes

- 1¾ pints (1 litre) full cream milk
- 6 eggs
- 1 vanilla pod
- 5oz (150 g) fructose
- 1 teaspoon cognac

- Bring the milk and split vanilla pod slowly to the boil. Allow to cool.
- In a mould, heat 2oz (50 g) of fructose with a little water to make a caramel.
- In a bowl, beat the eggs with the remaining 4oz (100 g) of fructose. Add the lukewarm milk little by little, beating all the time with the whisk. Add the cognac.
- Pour the mixture into the mould and cook for 45 minutes in a fairly hot oven at 200°C (400°F, gas mark 6) in a bain-marie. Allow to cool and then refrigerate for at least 4 hours.
- To turn out, place the mould for a few seconds in boiling water. Cover with a plate and turn over quickly. Alternatively, make and serve in individual ramekins.

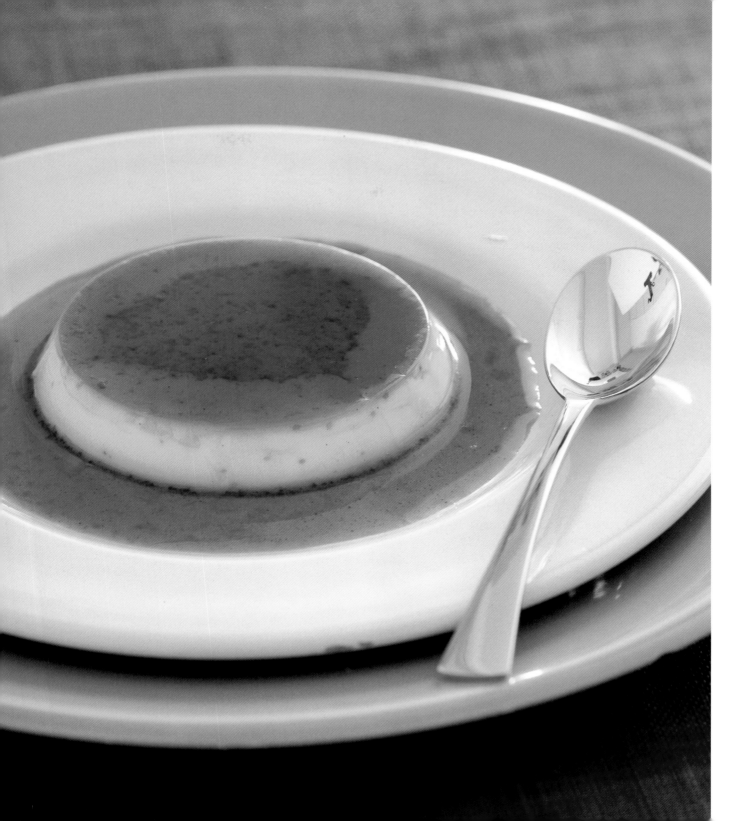

Catalan Cream with Fresh Raspberries Serves 4

Preparation: 10 minutes
Cooking time: 60 minutes
Refrigeration: 4 hours

- 1 punnet of raspberries
- 5 egg yolks
- 12oz (350 g) crème fraîche
- 5fl oz (15 cl) full cream milk
- 3oz (80 g) fructose
- 1 pinch cinnamon

- Bring the milk to the boil and then allow to cool for 10 minutes.
- Beat together egg yolks, fructose, and cinnamon. Whisk until the mixture turns white and creamy.
- Stir the milk and crème fraîche together and then add to the egg mixture, beating continuously.
- Cover the bottom of a shallow ovenproof dish or individual ramekins with raspberries and then pour the final mixture over the top.
- Place the shallow dish or ramekins in a hot bain-marie in a pre-heated oven at 130°C (260°F, gas mark ½) and cook for 55 minutes.
- Allow to cool to room temperature and refrigerate for at least 4 hours.
- Before serving, the catalan cream can be grilled for a few minutes until golden brown.

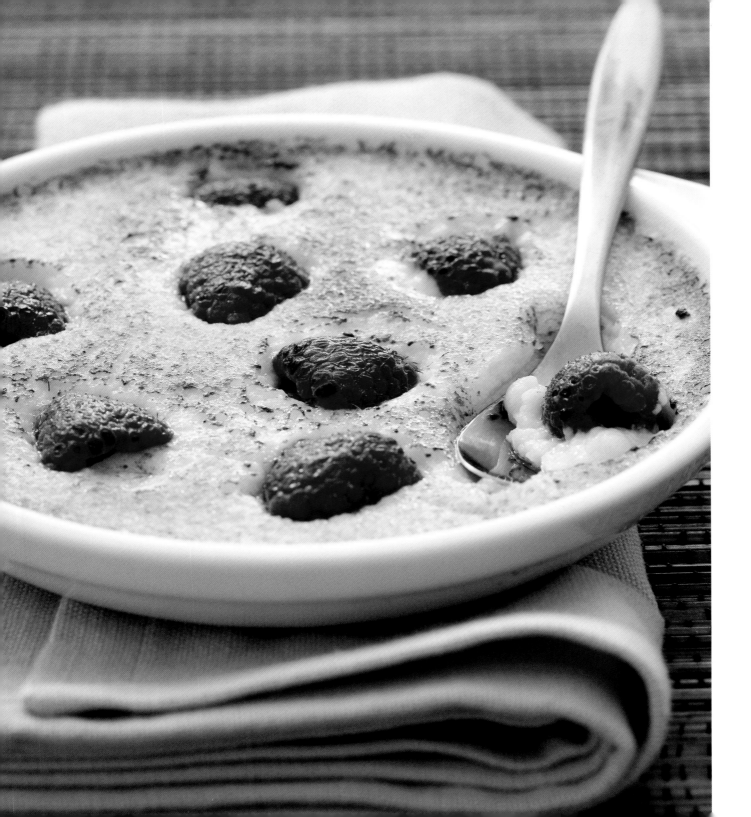

Whipped cream Nata

Serves 4

Preparation: 15 minutes
Refrigeration: 30 minutes

- 9fl oz (25 cl) whipping cream
- Vanilla essence
- 5oz (150 g) strawberries
- 5oz (150 g) raspberries
- 5oz (150 g) redcurrants
- 5oz (150 g) blackberries

- Put the cream and the bowl in which you are going to whip it in the freezer for 30 minutes.
- Prepare the fruits.
- Use an electric whisk to whip the cream until it is stiff (but be careful not to over-whip and turn it to butter).
- Before it is finished, add 2 or 3 drops of vanilla essence, whipping continuously.
- Place in the refrigerator and serve with summer fruits (strawberries, raspberries, redcurrants, blackberries).

Suggestions :
You can also add 1 or 2 tablespoons dark chocolate powder (Van Houten or similar) towards the end, when the cream is almost whipped. In hot weather, whip the cream with the bowl placed in a larger one containing ice cubes.

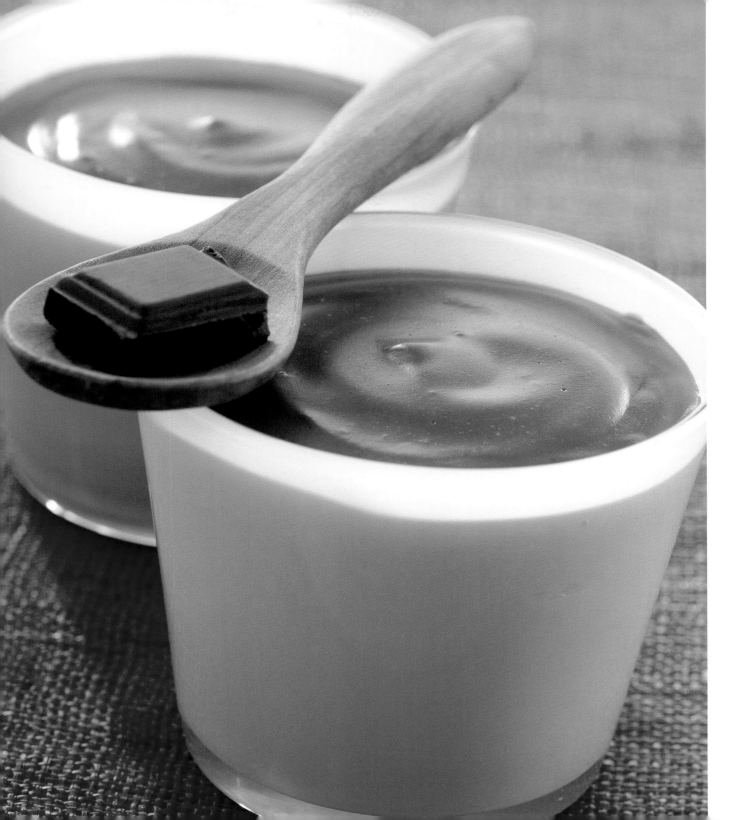

Coconut flan

Serves 4

Preparation: 10 minutes
Cooking time: 45 minutes

- 5 eggs
- 4oz (100 g) grated coconut
- 4oz (100 g) fructose
- 14fl oz (40 cl) whipping cream

- In a bowl, beat the eggs together with the fructose. Add the whipping cream.
Then add the coconut.
- Pour into a 1 litre (2 pint) cake tin, cover with a cloth and allow to rest for 15 minutes.
- Cook for 45 minutes in a bain-marie in the oven at 130°C (260°F, gas mark ½). Check that the flan is set (insert a skewer into the middle and it should come out clean).
- Remove from the oven and allow to cool to room temperature (or until cold) before serving with a raspberry coulis or hot chocolate sauce.

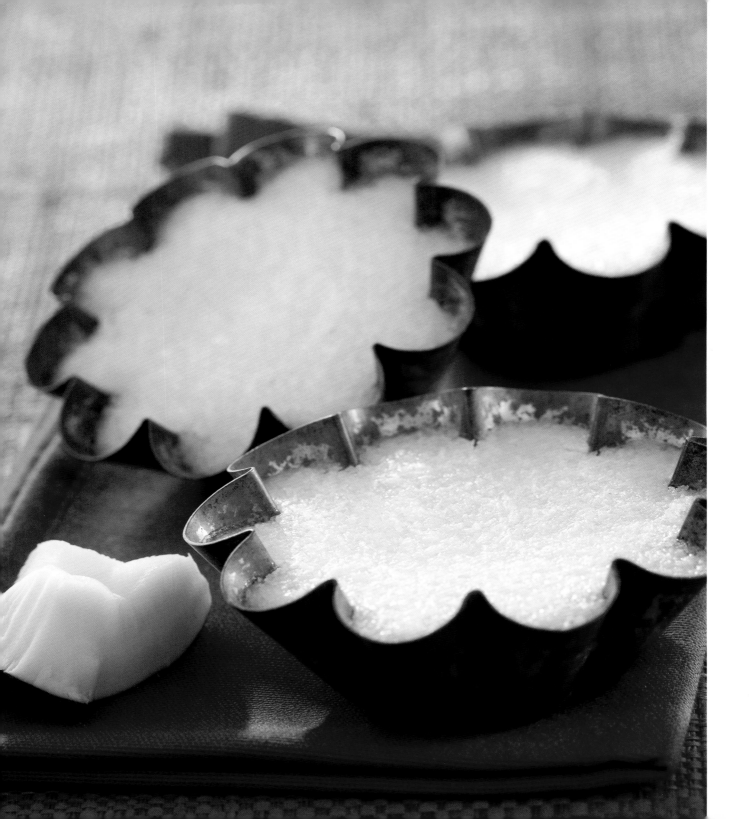

Strawberries with orange and mint Serves 4

Preparation: 10 minutes
Cooking time: 15 minutes

- 1lb (500 g) strawberries
- 3 oranges
- ½ glass cointreau
- 2oz (50 g) fructose
- 12 leaves of mint

- Squeeze the juice out of the oranges.
- Put the orange juice, Cointreau, fructose and 5 chopped mint leaves into a small pan.
Bring to the boil and reduce by half. Allow to cool.
- Rinse the strawberries under the tap and drain on kitchen paper.
- Remove the stalks and cut in two.
- Arrange in individual plates.
- Coat with the minted syrup of orange.
- Decorate with the remaining mint leaves and serve.

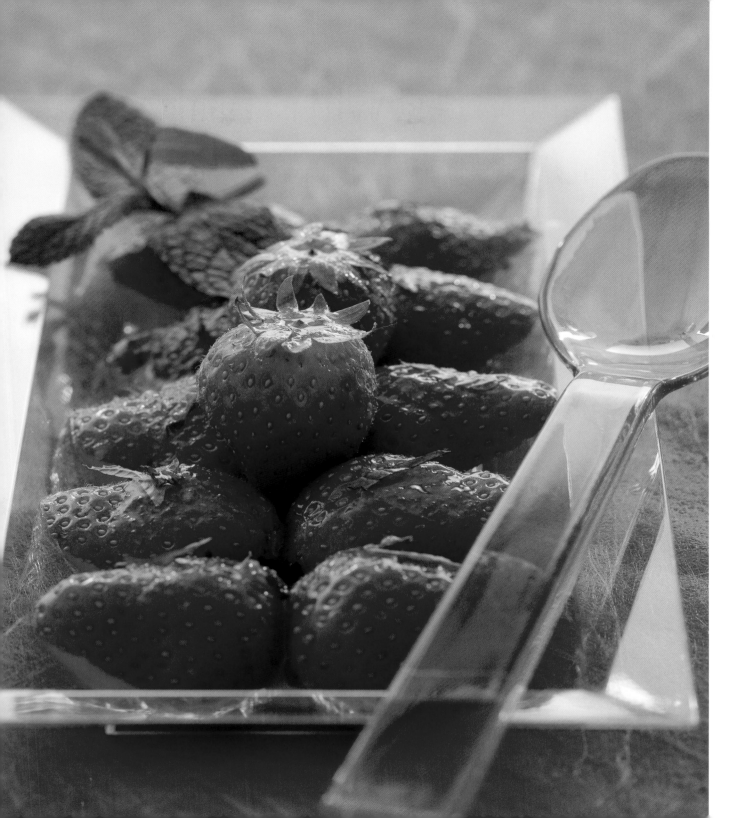

Strawberries with mint and yoghurt Serves 4 to 5

Preparation: 10 minutes

- 26oz (750 g) strawberries
- 3 natural yoghurts
- 1 large bunch of mint
- 2 tablespoons of sugar-free strawberry jam

- Rinse the strawberries under the tap and drain on kitchen paper. Remove all stalks. Arrange in small bowls.
- Remove the mint leaves from their stems and chop finely.
- In a bowl, mix the yoghurt, chopped mint and strawberry jam. Chill in the fridge.
- Pour over the strawberries and serve.

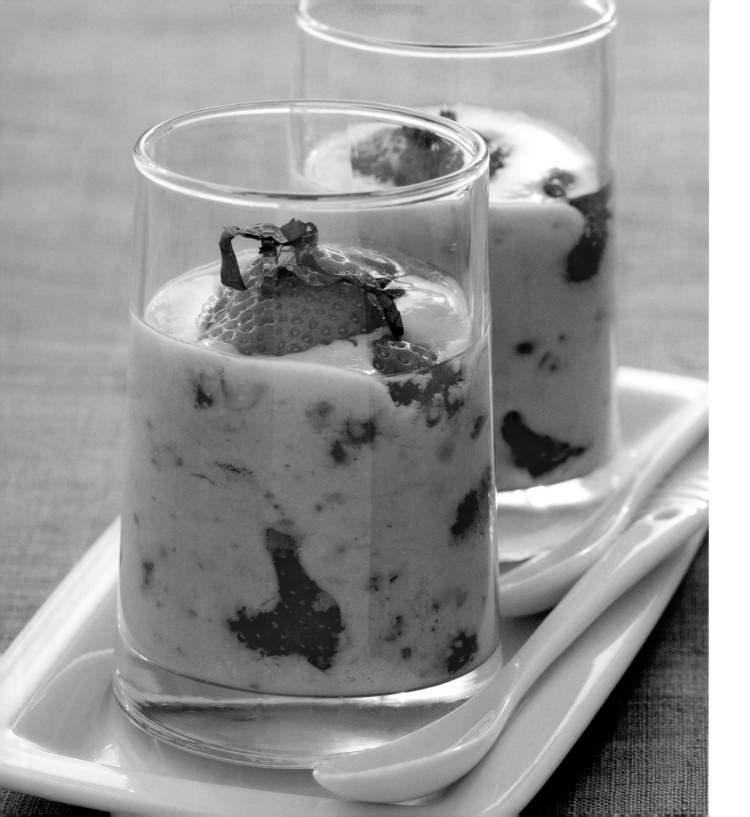

Raspberry bush

Serves 4 to 5

Preparation: 20 minutes
Cooking time: 20 minutes
Refrigeration: 5 to 6 hours

- 9oz (250 g) raspberries
- 4 egg yolks
- 18fl oz (50 cl) full cream milk
- 2 tablespoons fructose
- 1 vanilla pod
- 4 leaves of gelatine (or equivalent of agar-agar)
- 7fl oz (20 cl) whipping cream

- Split the vanilla pod with a knife and add to the milk. Bring the milk slowly to the boil and allow to cool for 10 minutes. Discard the pod.
- Beat the egg yolks and pour in the milk gradually while continuing to whisk.
- Return the mixture to a pan over a very low heat (preferably a bain-marie) and allow to thicken slightly. Stir constantly with a whisk. Add the fructose.
- Soak the leaves of gelatine in cold water for a few minutes. Squeeze out and add to the egg mixture, mixing in well with the whisk so that the gelatine dissolves completely. Place on one side and allow to cool for 1 hour.
- Whip the cream and fold into the egg mixture before it sets.
- Pour the mixture into moulds together with the raspberries.
- Cover with plastic film and place in the fridge for at least 5 or 6 hours.
- Serve plain or with whipped cream, sprinkled with cocoa or grated chocolate.

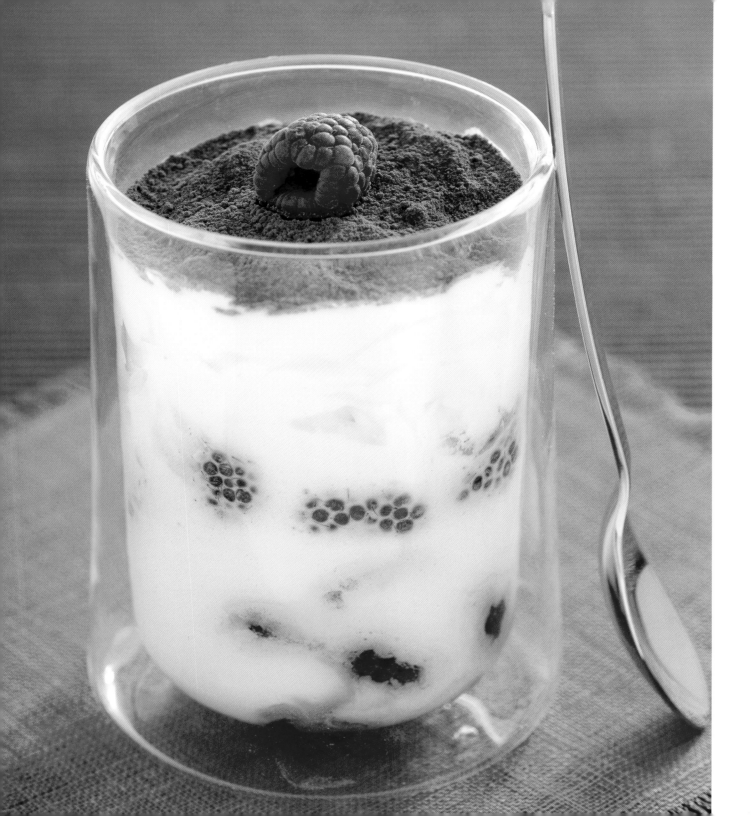

Red fruit in red wine jelly

Serves 6

Preparation: 20 minutes
Cooking time: 10 minutes
Refrigeration: 8 to 10 hours

- 7oz (200 g) strawberries
- 7oz (200 g) raspberries
- 3½ oz (100 g) blueberries
- 3½ oz (100 g) blackberries
- 14fl oz (40 cl) red wine with high tannin content, like Corbières, Côtes du Rhône . . .
- 4fl oz (10 cl) liquid fructose (or 4 tablespoons)
- ½ teaspoon cinnamon
- 7 leaves of gelatine (or the equivalent of agar-agar)
- Mint leaves

- Place a fluted mould in the freezer.
- Pour the wine into a pan and add the cinnamon. Bring to the boil and remove immediately from the heat.
- Meanwhile, prepare the fruit.
- Soften the gelatine for 5 minutes in cold water. Squeeze out and then dissolve in the warm wine. Add the liquid fructose. Stir well and allow to cool.
- Take the mould out of the freezer and coat the inside with the wine jelly by tipping the mould from side to side, making sure no part is left uncovered by the jelly.
- Return the mould to the freezer for a few minutes and repeat the coating operation until the jelly lining is about 1cm thick (just under ½ in) all over.
- Turn the fruit into the mould. Spread out well using a spoon or spatula and layer of mint leaves.
- Pour the rest of the wine jelly carefully over the top and cover with aluminium foil.
- Leave in the fridge overnight or for at least 8 or 10 hours.
- Unmould just prior to serving.

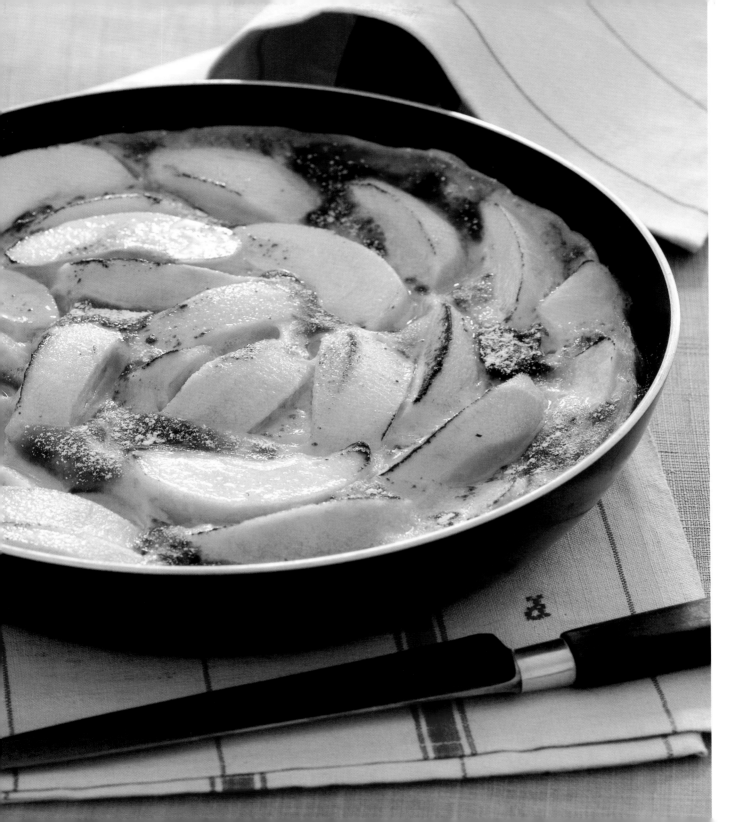

Rich chocolate cake with roasted pistachios

Serves 4

Preparation: 15 minutes
Cooking time: 35 minutes

- 3 egg yolks + 3 egg whites
- 3oz (80 g) fructose
- 4fl oz (12 cl) olive oil (or sunflower oil)
- 4oz (120 g) powder almonds
- 7oz (200 g) dark chocolate with
70 % minimum cocoa solids
- 3½ oz (100 g) roasted pistachios (chopped)

For the custard (optional)
- 5 egg yolks
- 3oz (80 g) fructose
- 18oz (500 ml) skimmed milk
- 2 vanilla pods

- Preheat the oven to 150°C (300°F, gas mark 2).
- In a bowl, beat the egg yolks together with the fructose. Add the melted chocolate and the oil. Stir well.
- Fold the almonds and the half pistachios into the mixture. Reserve.
- Beat the whites, adding a pinch of salt, until they form stiff peaks. Fold the whites carefully into the chocolate mixture with a metal spoon.
- Transfer the mixture to a cake tin (oiled) and sprinkle with the other half of pistachios.
- Put to the oven and cook for 30 to 35 minutes.

For the custard (optional)
- Boil the milk with the vanilla pod.
- In a bowl, beat the egg yolks together with the fructose.
Add the lukewarm milk and whisk vigorously.
- Place on a low heat again for 3 minutes to thicken.
- Leave in the fridge for several hours.

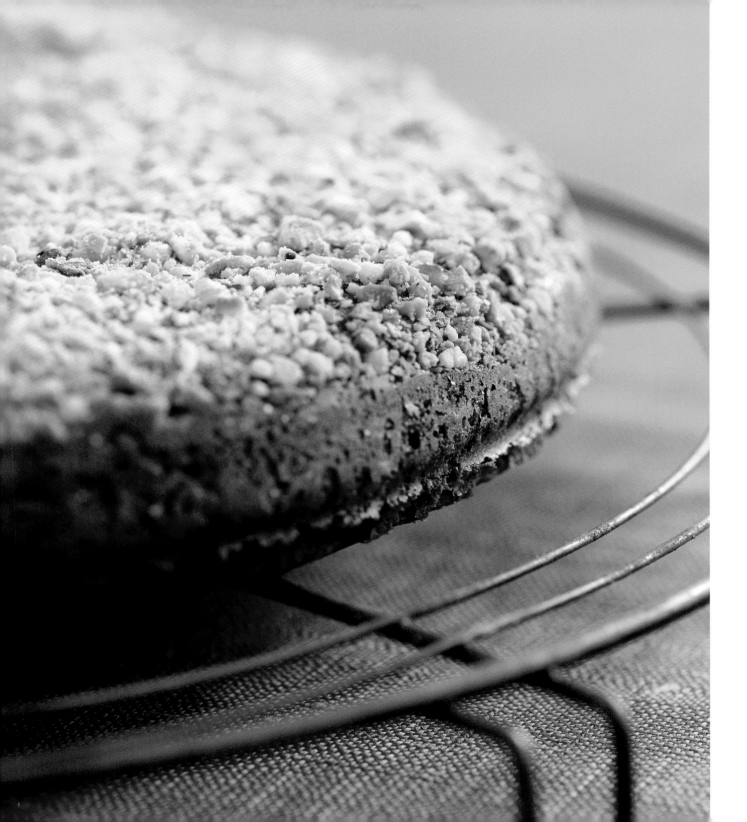

Baked summer fruits dessert Serves 8

Preparation: 10 minutes
Cooking time: 25/30 minutes

- 26oz (750 g) strawberries
- 26oz (750 g) raspberries
- 5 eggs
- 18fl oz (50 cl) semi-skimmed milk
- 7oz (200 ml) low-fat crème fraîche
- 4 tablespoons fructose

- Cut the strawberries in half.
- In a gratin dish place alternately layers of strawberries and raspberries, with each layer separated by a thin layer of crème fraîche.
- Finish with a layer of raspberries.
- Lightly beat the eggs and add the milk and fructose.
- Pour the mixture over the fruit and bake at 200°C (400°F, gas mark 6) for 25 to 30 minutes.
- Serve lukewarm or cold.

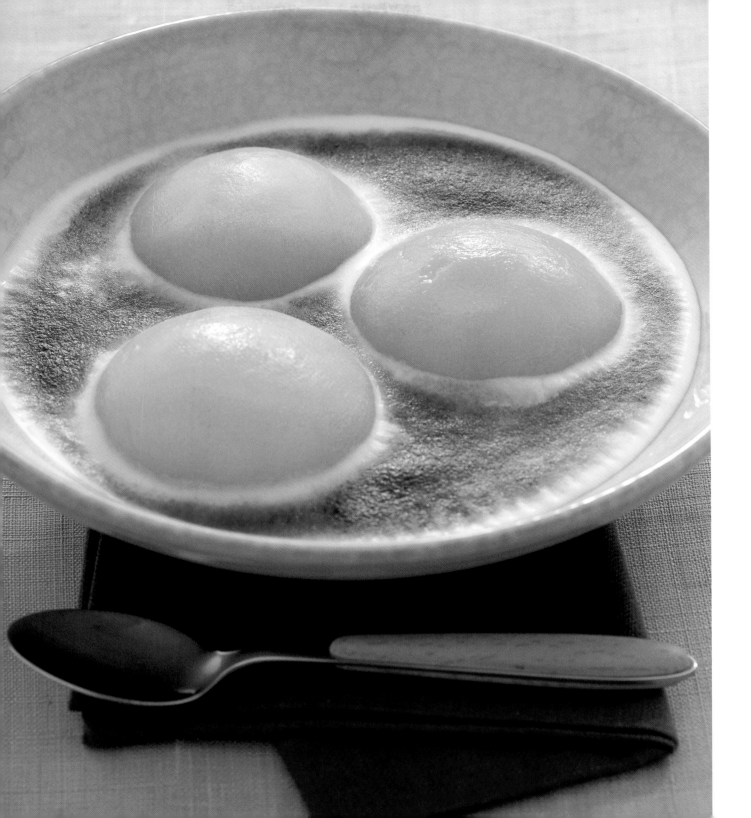

Grilled pear zabaglione

Serves 4

Preparation: 20 minutes
Cooking time: 35 minutes

- 8 good-sized pears
- 3½ oz (100 g) fructose
- 5 egg yolks
- Juice of 1 orange
- 1 teaspoon vanilla extract
- 1 tablespoon rum
- Mint leaves

- Peel the pears, quarter and remove the cores.
- Slice each quarter into two.
- Arrange the pear slices on the bottom of an ovenware dish lightly brushed with oil. Sprinkle 1oz
(20 g) fructose over the top.
- Place under the grill for 5 to 10 minutes, to allow the pears to brown lightly without burning. Reserve.
- To make the sabayon, whisk the egg yolks and fructose together until they begin to turn slightly
white and creamy.
- Add the orange juice, vanilla, rum, and cooking juice from the pears.
- Cook gently in a bain-marie, beating constantly, until the cream thickens slightly.
- Arrange the pear slices on serving plates. Pour the cream over the top and decorate with a mint leaf.

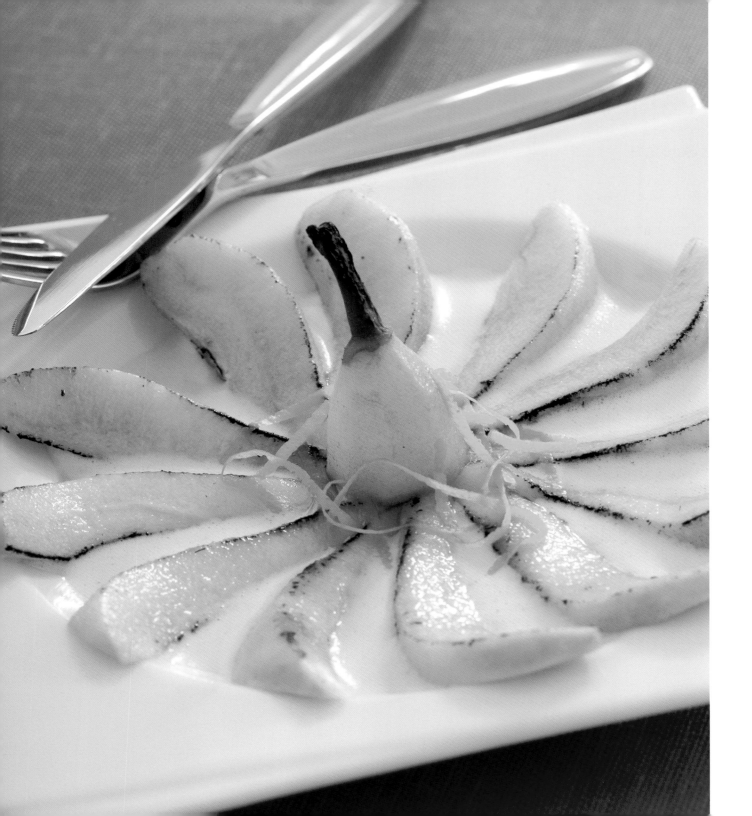

Chocolate macaroons

Serves 6

Preparation: 20 minutes
Cooking time: 5 minutes

- 6 egg whites
- 3½ oz (100 g) fructose
- 6oz (180 g) almonds (shell)
- 2oz (50 g) almonds powder
- Olive oil

For the ganache
- 11oz (300 g) dark chocolate with 70 % minimum cocoa solids
- 2oz (50 g) low fat crème fraîche
- Unsweetened cocoa powder

- Preheat the oven to 250°C (500°F, gas mark 8/9).
- Blend the fructose with the almonds (powder and shell).
- Beat the egg whites until they form stiff peaks.
- Fold gently into the almond mixture, a little at a time.
- Grease the oven pan with oil.
- Spread the mixture using a pastry bag (or by the help of circles that can be filled) to form galettes 5 to 12 cm in diameter.
- Cook for 5 to 7 minutes. Keep watch over the cooking. Remove gently with a spatula and set aside.

For the ganache:
- Melt the chocolate in a bain-marie. Add the crème fraîche.
- Whip vigorously and remove from the heat.
- Soak the macaroons into the chocolate.
- Allow to cool and sprinkle with cocoa. Then refrigerate for 1 to 2 hours.

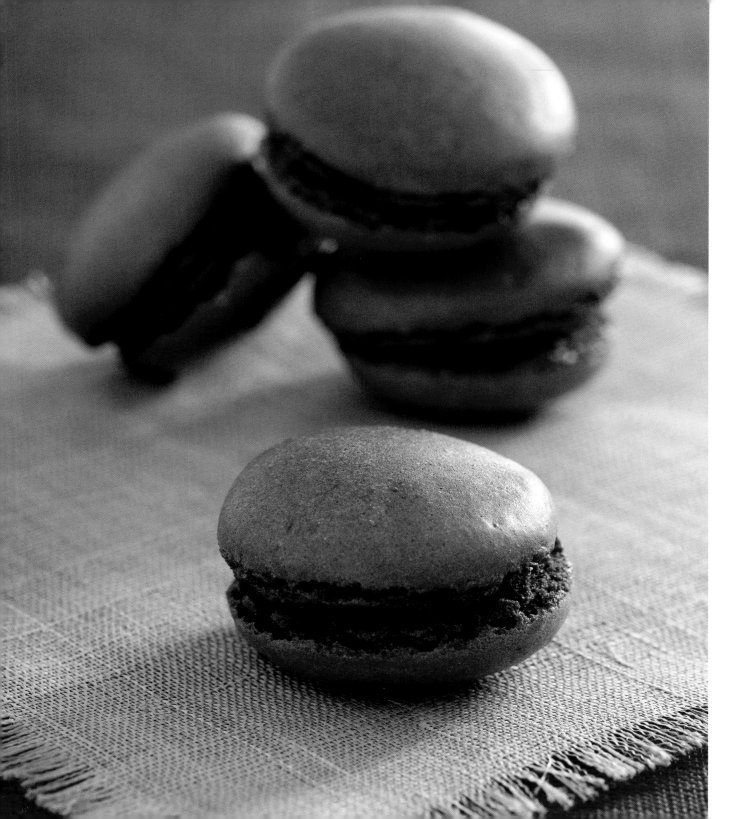

Rich chocolate dessert

Serves 4

Preparation: 20 minutes
Cooking time: 10 minutes

- 9oz (250 g) dark chocolate with 70 % minimum cocoa solids
- 5 eggs
- 1/2 glass milk
- 1 pinch salt

- Melt 200 g (7oz) of the chocolate in a bain-marie with the half glass of milk.
- Separate the eggs.
- Beat the whites, adding a pinch of salt, until they form stiff peaks. Add the yolks, beating continuously with an electric whisk until the mixture is smooth.
- Add this mixture to the chocolate, still in the bain-marie. Stir continuously until the mixture turns thick and 'lumpy' (as the eggs cook, the mixture will shrink in volume and will take on a consistency like scrambled eggs).
- Transfer the mixture to a cake tin or shallow dish which will allow for it to be spread to 2 cm (1in) deep, and allow to cool a little.
- Meanwhile, melt the remaining 2oz (50 g) of dark chocolate in a bain-marie, with 4 or 5 tablespoons of water.
- When it is completely melted, pour over the cake, spreading it like icing, using a spatula.
- This rich chocolate dessert can be eaten right away, lukewarm, or cold after 1 hour in the refrigerator. It can also be eaten with whipped cream.

Recommandation:
If you keep it in the fridge for a while, remove 2 hours before serving.

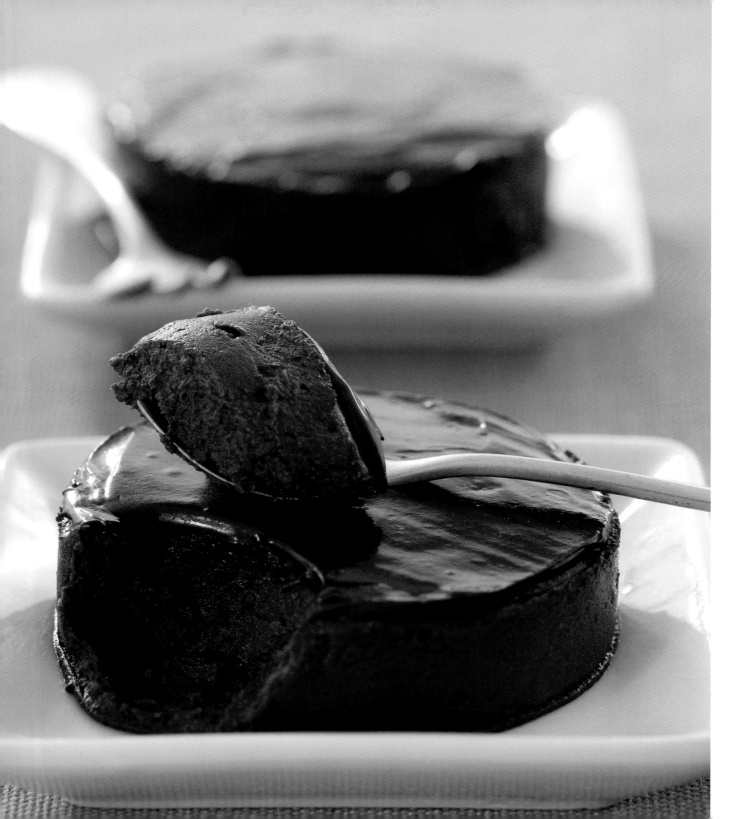

Apricot mousse

Serves 4

Preparation: 15 minutes
Refrigeration: 1 hour

- 1lb (500 g) apricots
- 1 lemon
- 2 tablespoons fructose
- 2 leaves (two thirds of sachet) of gelatine
- 5oz (150 g) fromage frais (20 % fat)
- 3½ oz (100 g) low-fat cream

- Blanch the apricots in boiling water for 1 minute.
- Drain, skin and cut in half to remove the stone.
- Blend to a purée and add the lemon juice and the fructose.
- If using gelatine leaves, soften in cold water and drain. Melt the gelatine in 2 tablespoons water in a bain-marie and immediately combine with the apricot purée.
- Whip the fromage frais and add to the mixture, combining thoroughly.
- Pour the mousse into ramekins and set in the refrigerator for 3 hours.
- Serve well chilled.

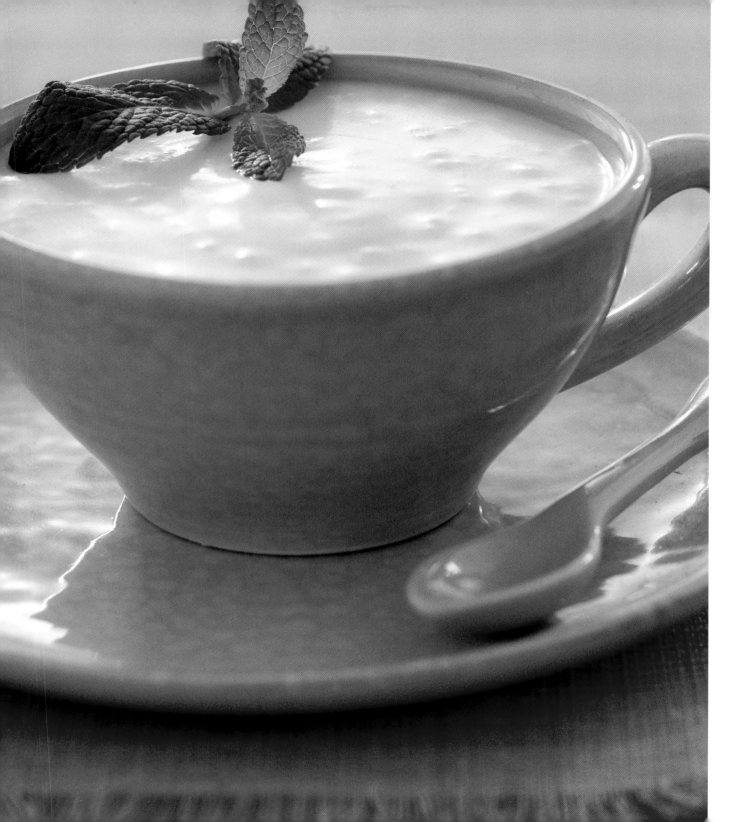

Brazilian mousse

Serves 6

Preparation: 20 minutes
Cooking time: 10 minutes
Refrigeration: 5 to 6 hours

- 4 tablespoons instant coffee
- 7fl oz (20 cl) whipping cream
- 6 eggs
- 3 leaves of gelatine (or the equivalent of agar-agar)
- ½ glass rum
- 3½ oz (100 g) fructose

- In a bain-marie, dissolve the instant coffee in the rum and cream. Add the fructose and dissolve.
- Immerse the gelatine in cold water for a few minutes. Remove and squeeze out. Add to the coffee mixture and dissolve. Allow to cool.
- Break the eggs and separate the whites from the yolks.
- Add a pinch of salt to the whites and whisk until very stiff.
- Mix the coffee cream with the egg yolks. Fold the whites carefully into the coffee mixture with a metal spoon.
- Transfer to a glass serving bowl, or 6 individual small moulds.
- Put in a fridge for 5 to 6 hours.
- Before serving, sprinkle with freshly ground coffee beans.

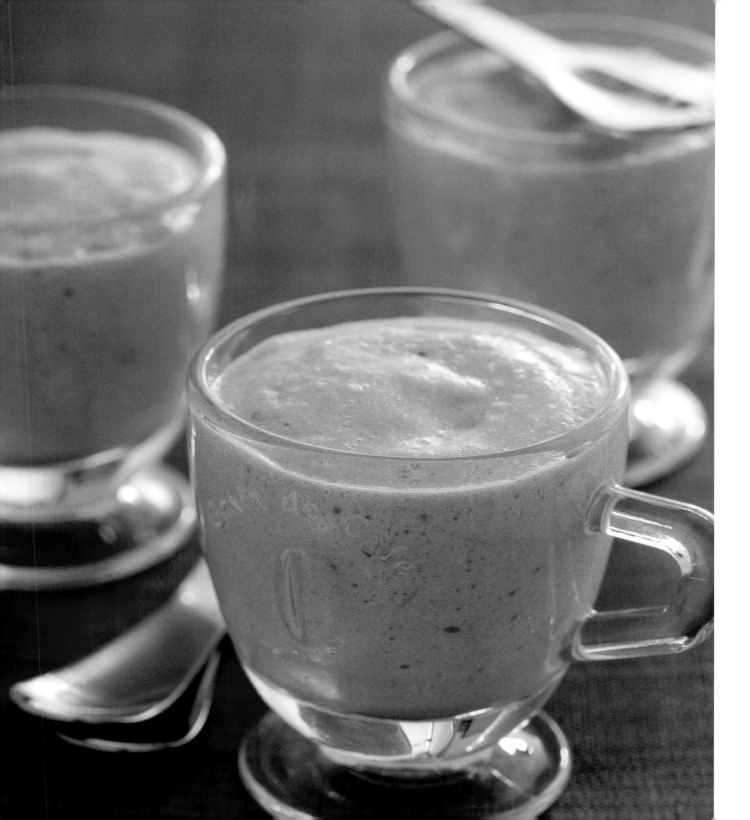

Chocolate mousse

Serves 6 to 8

Preparation: 25 minutes
Cooking time: 10 minutes
Refrigeration: 5 hours

- 14oz (400 g) dark chocolate with 70 % minimum cocoa solids
- 8 eggs
- 1/2 glass rum (70 ml)
- 4 teaspoons instant coffee
- 1 pinch salt

- Break the chocolate into pieces and place in a bain-marie.
- Make half a cup of very strong coffee and add to the chocolate, together with the rum.
- Melt the chocolate in the bain-marie, stirring with a spatula.
- Separate the eggs and beat the whites, with a pinch of salt added, until they form stiff peaks.
- Allow the chocolate to cool down a little in a large bowl and add the egg yolks, stirring briskly.
- Gently fold in the beaten egg whites, a little at a time, to obtain a smooth mousse.
- Allow to set in the refrigerator for at least 5 hours before serving.

Suggestion:
The addition of orange zest will add a delightful flavour to this mousse.

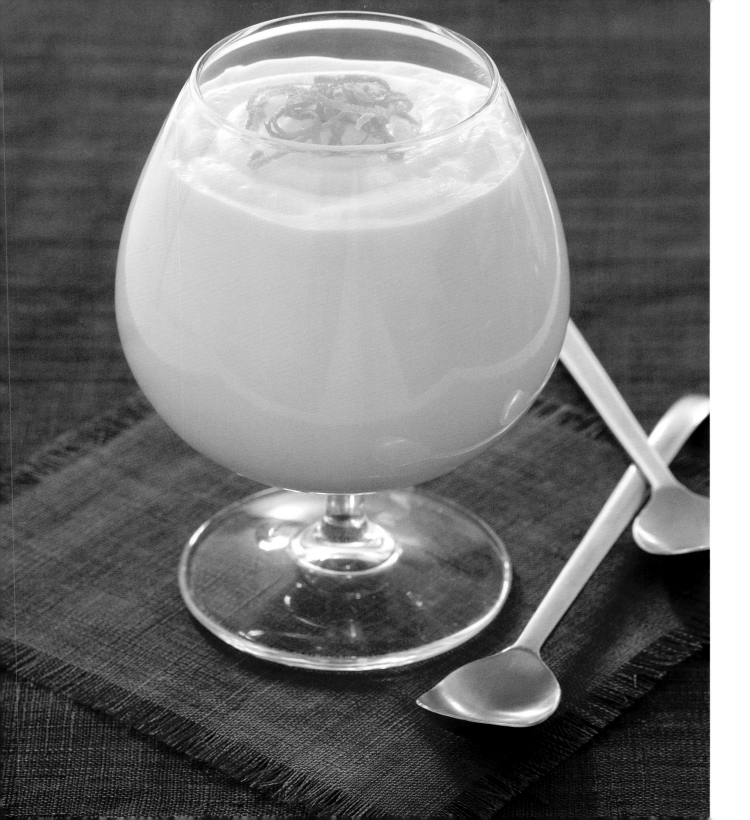

Fresh almond mousse

Serves 4 to 5

Preparation: 25 minutes
Cooking time: 15 minutes
Refrigeration: 4 hours

- 4 eggs
- 3½ oz (100 g) freshly peeled almonds
- 12fl oz (35 cl) very cold whipping cream
- 3½ oz (100 g) red currants
- 3½ oz (100 g) fructose
- Juice of ½ lemon
- 1 teaspoon lemon zest
- 1 tablespoon liquid fructose
- Mint leaves to decorate

- Break the eggs into a bowl and whisk with the fructose in a bain-marie over a low heat. Continue beating till the mixture becomes firm and frothy.
- Remove from the bain-marie and continue whisking until the mixture has cooled. Add the lemon juice, the liquid fructose and then the lemon zest. When fully mixed, place on one side and reserve.
- Wash the red currants, remove the stalks, and dry on kitchen paper.
- Chop the almonds. Over a low heat, lightly brown in a dry non-stick pan.
- Whisk the cream until stiff. Fold in the egg mixture and then carefully add the red currants and chopped almonds.
- Line the inside of a fluted mould with plastic film. Pour in the mixture and wrap the film over the top.
- Place in the fridge for 4 hours.
- Unmould onto a plate. Decorate with mint leaves and serve.

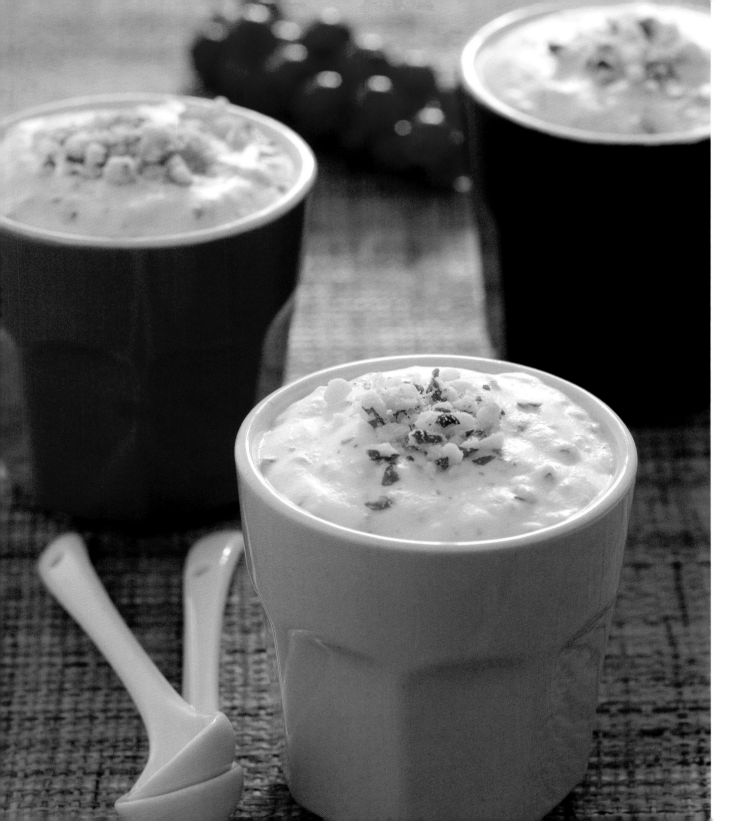

Floating islands

Serves 6 to 8

Preparation: 30 minutes
Cooking time: 30 minutes

- 1 vanilla pod
- 8 eggs
- 1¾ pints (1 litre) semi-skimmed milk
- 3 tablespoons fructose
- 1 pinch salt

- Separate the eggs. Beat the whites until they form stiff peaks, adding a pinch of salt.
- Boil the milk with the vanilla pod and half a glass of water. Keep it just simmering.
- Use a tablespoon to scoop up "snowballs" of beaten egg white and place on the surface of the milk. Poach them for 1 minute each side, remove and drain on a clothe
- Make an egg custard by beating the egg yolks and adding the lukewarm milk. (Dilute slightly to make the quantity up to 1 litre.) Whisk vigorously.
- Place on a low heat again to thicken. Sweeten with the fructose at the last minute.
- Allow to cool. Serve with the 'snowballs' floating on the custard.

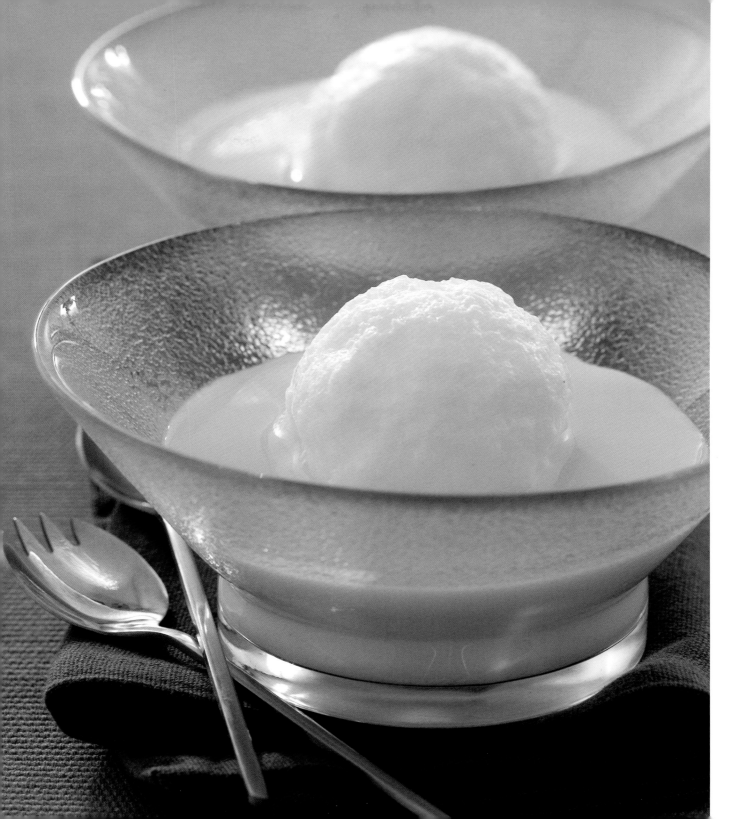

Egg custards

Serves 5

Preparation: 10 minutes
Cooking time: 30 minutes
Refrigeration: 3 hours

- 1 pint (50 cl) semi-skimmed milk
- 5 egg yolks
- 2 tablespoons fructose
- 1 vanilla pod

- Heat the milk with the vanilla pod, let it cool slightly and remove the vanilla pod.
- Beat the egg yolks vigorously and pour the lukewarm milk over. Add the fructose and pour the mixture into ramekins.
- Cook in a bain-marie in a moderate oven at 180°C (350°, gas mark 3-4) for about 30 minutes.
- Serve cold in the ramekins.

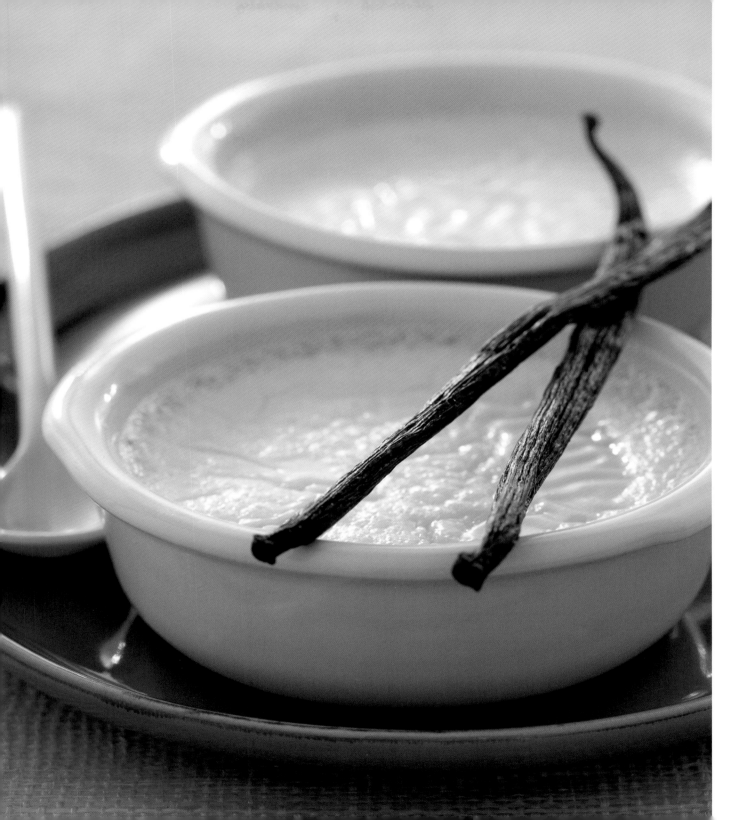

Papaya with blueberries

Serves 4

Preparation: 10 minutes
Refrigeration: 1 à 3 hours

- 1 big (or 2 small) papaya
- 5oz (150 g) blueberries
- 2oz (50 g) fructose
- ½ lemon
- Mint leaves

- Cut in half the papaya.
- Remove the seed and collect the flesh.
- In a bowl, dice the flesh.
- Add the blueberries and stir well.
- Add the lemon juice and the fructose. Stir well and set in the refrigerator for 1 to 3 hours.

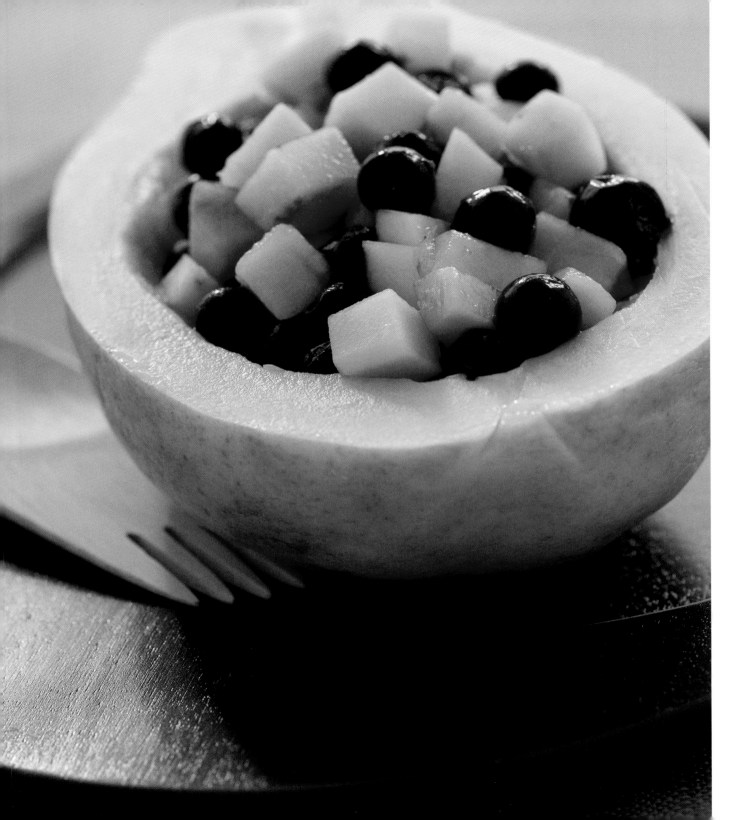

Chick-pea pancake (soca)

Makes 1 pancake

Preparation: 10 minutes
Cooking time: 6-7 minutes

- 9oz (250 g) chick-pea flour
- 18fl oz (50 cl) water
- 6 teaspoons olive oil
- 1½ teaspoon salt

- In a large mixing-bowl, add the cold water to the chick-pea flour with 1 teaspoon olive oil.
Salt and put to the mixer. Liquidize.
- Put the pan on the heat and add the olive oil. Don't let it smoke.
- Pour the mixture and mix actively with the hot oil.
- Cook for 6 to 7 minutes. The cooking is finished when the oil and water are completely absorbed
and don't boil on the surface.
- Eventually, put the pan over the grill for 1 or 2 minutes to make the top golden-brown.

Suggestion:
The Soca can be used as a base to make a Montignac pizza. It can also be eaten as a crepe, or
used as a substitute to bread (very low GI) and used to spread tuna or goose rillettes, sprinkled
with a little pepper.

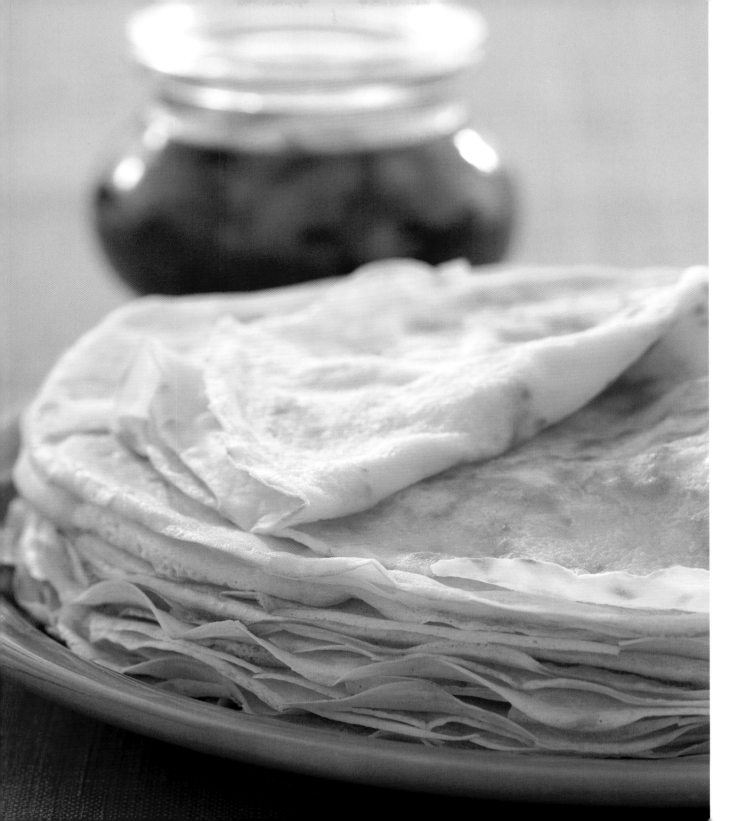

Peaches with cheese and raspberries Serves 4

Preparation: 10 minutes
Cooking time: 10 minutes

- 1lb (500 g) fromage frais – strained
- 2 tablespoons crème fraîche
- 6 good-size peaches
- 3½ oz (100 g) sugar-free raspberry jam
- Mint leaves

- Poach the peaches for about 10 minutes. Peel, halve and remove the stones.
- Liquidize the fromage frais, crème fraîche and raspberry jam. Pour into the bottom of individual dipped plates.
- Arrange 3 peach halves on top of each plate. Cover with plastic film and place in the fridge.
- Serve chilled and decorate with mint.

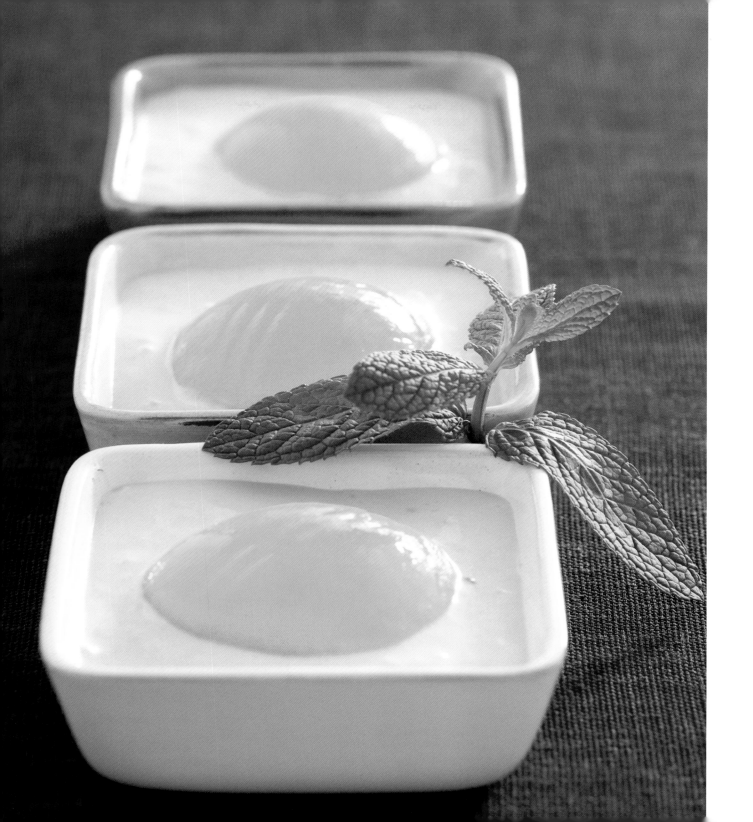

Mango sorbet

Serves 4

Preparation: 10 minutes
Refrigeration: 3 hours

- 2 ripe mangoes (providing 16oz or 450 g flesh)
- 1 small tin of condensed unsweetened semi-skimmed milk (3½ oz or 100 g)
- 2 tablespoons lemon juice
- A few drops vanilla essence
- 2 tablespoons fructose

- Peel and stone the mangoes and chop the flesh into small pieces.
- Blend with the concentrated milk, the lemon juice, vanilla essence and fructose (the consistency should be light and frothy).
- Place the mousse in the freezer for about 3 hours. Use a scoop to serve, as if it were ice-cream.

Recommandation:
Use a sorbet-maker for best results.

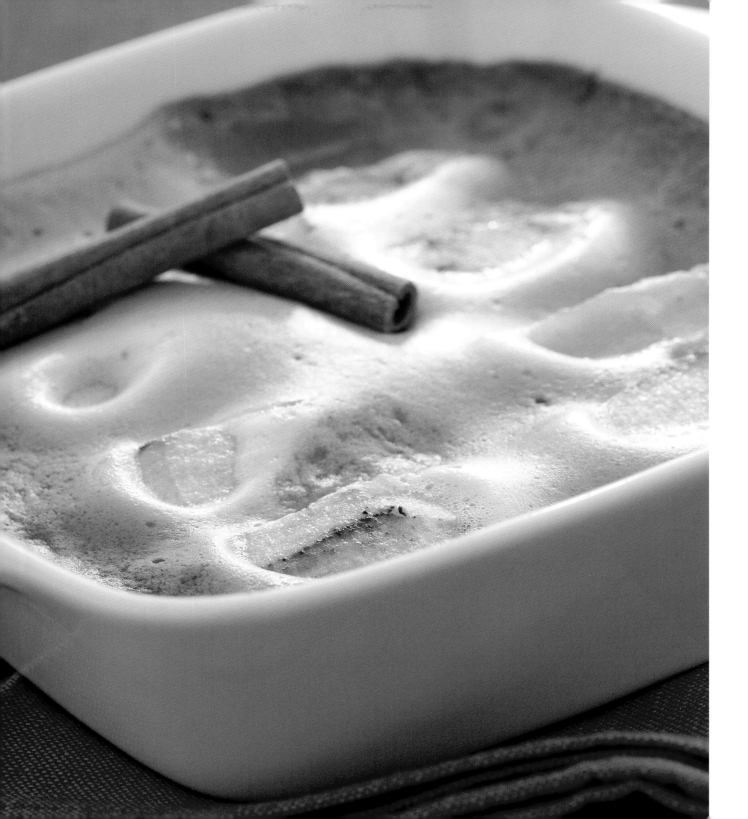

Apricots and custard

Serves 4

Preparation: 15 minutes
Cooking time: 20 minutes

- 20 apricots
- 2 tablespoons fructose
- ½ glass rum
- 8 egg yolks
- 1¾ pints (1 litre) milk
- 3 tablespoons fructose
- 1 vanilla pod
- sugar-free cocoa powder

- Split open the apricots and remove the stones.
- Place in a steamer skin-side facing downwards. Sprinkle with 2 tablespoons of fructose and cook for 10 minutes. Allow to drain. Flambé with the rum and allow to cool. Reserve in the fridge.
- Split the vanilla pod with a knife and add to the milk. Slowly bring the milk to the boil. Remove from the heat and allow to cool for 10 minutes.
- Beat the egg yolks, adding the warm milk slowly to the mixture. Then whisk briskly.
- Return the mixture to a low heat to thicken (preferably in a bain-marie), beating constantly. When the custard has the right consistency, allow to cool for a few minutes and add fructose.
- Leave in the fridge for several hours.
- To serve, place 8 to 10 apricot halves in a shallow dish. Ladle custard over the top and dust with the cocoa powder.

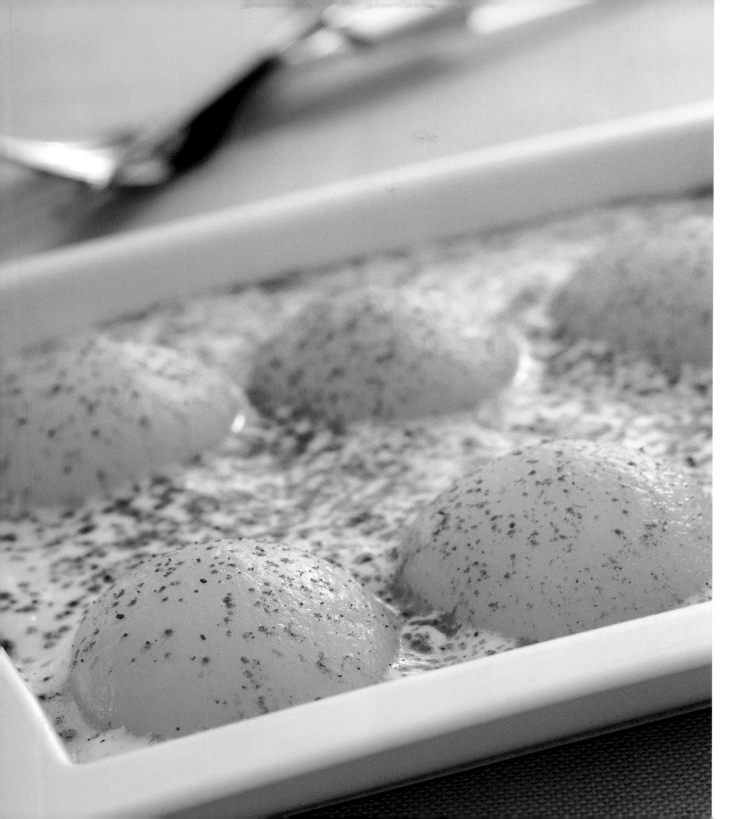

Mango and raspberry soup with mint

Serves 4

Preparation: 20 minutes
Refrigeration: 2 to 3 hours

- 2-3 ripe mangoes
- 14oz (400 g) fresh raspberries
- 3½ oz (100 g) fructose
- About thirty mint leaves
- ½fl oz (1 cl) Cognac (optional)

- Make syrup with the fructose and water. Add the Cognac.
- Peel and stone the mangoes and slice.
- Remove about twenty mint leaves from their stems and chop finely.
- Arrange the fruits (mango slices and raspberries) on 4 serving plates.
- Pour the syrup over the top and sprinkle with chopped mint.
- Decorate with mint leaves.
- Cover with plastic film and place in the fridge for 2 to 3 hours.

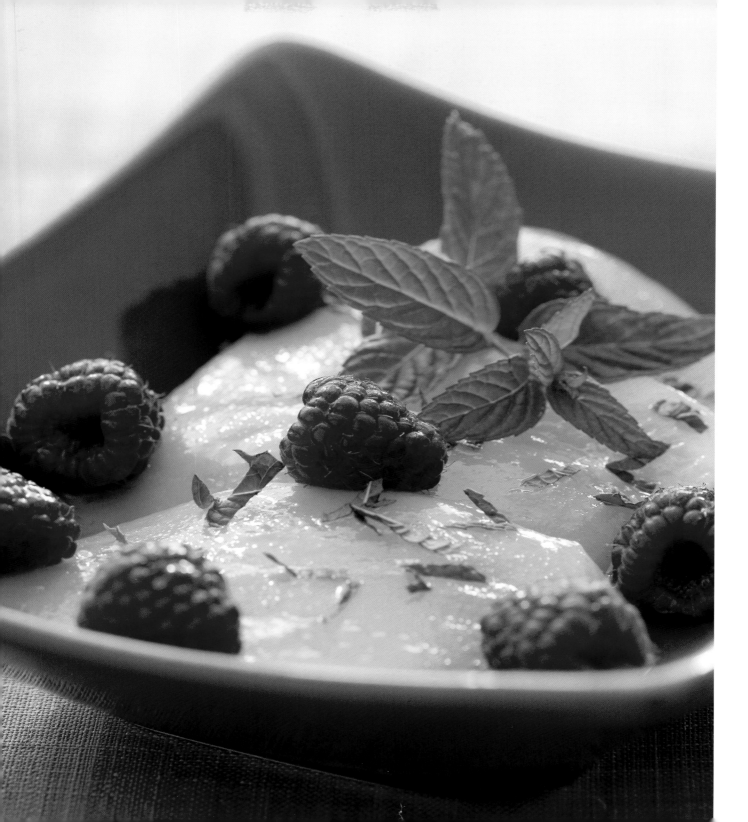

Peach and apple soup with cinnamon

Serves 4

Preparation: 20 minutes
Cooking time: 25 minutes

- 3¼ lb (1.5 kg) yellow peaches
- 28oz (800 g) apples
- 2oz (50 g) fructose
- 1 tablespoon cinnamon
- 1 yogurt with 0% fat
- 1 sachet of shelled walnuts

- Peel the peaches and the apples and quarter.
- In a boiler, pour 3 tablespoons water and add the fruits.
- Sprinkle with cinnamon and fructose. Stir well.
- Cover and cook on a low heat for about 25 minutes.
- Before serving, collect and reduce the cook juice in a high heat to make syrup.
- Mix the syrup with the yogurt.
- Arrange the fruits (peaches and apples) on 4 serving plates.
- Pour the syrup over the top and sprinkle with shelled walnuts.
- Serve lukewarm.

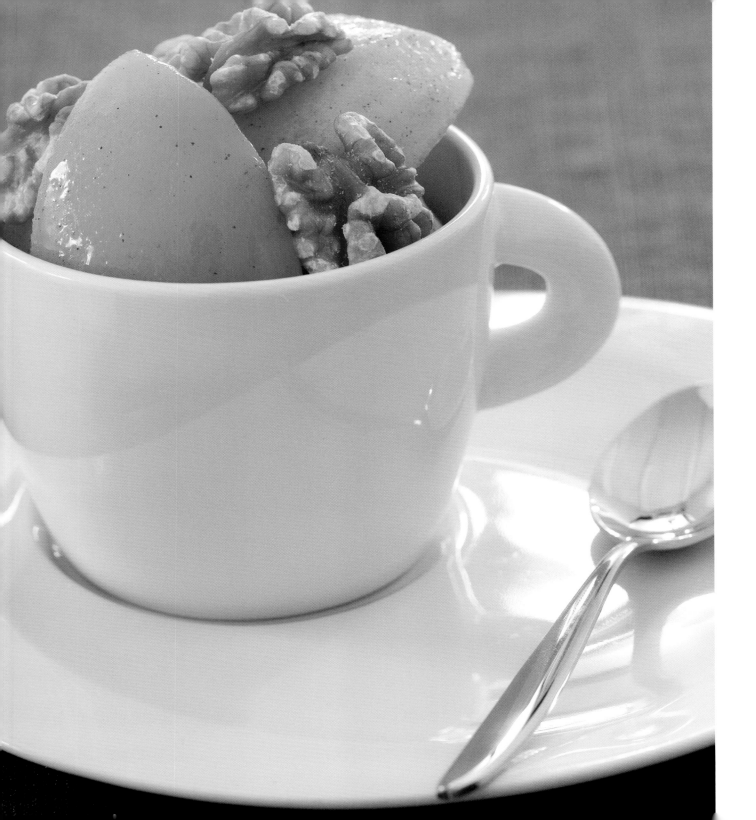

Upside-down apple tart

Serves 4

Preparation: 30 minutes
Cooking time: 25 minutes

- 3 eggs + 1 yolk egg
- 2¼ lb (1 kg) apples
- 5oz (150 g) fructose
- 5oz (150 g) almonds powder
- Olive oil

- Preheat the oven to 200°C (400°F, gas mark 5).
- Peel, core and quarter the apples.
- In the pan, cook gently the apples with a little of olive oil for 10 minutes and stir continuously.
- Sprinkle with ¾ of the fructose and allow to caramelise a little.
- Oil a cake mould.
- Arrange the apple quarters on the bottom of the mould.
- Break the eggs into a bowl. Add the yolk and the fructose. Beat together. Add the almonds powder.
- Pour the mixture onto the apples.
- Put in the oven and cook for 12 to 15 minutes.
- Remove from the oven and allow to cool 20 minutes.
- Turn over the mould on a big plate and leave the mould on the top for at least 30 minutes.
- Turn out from the mould just before serving.

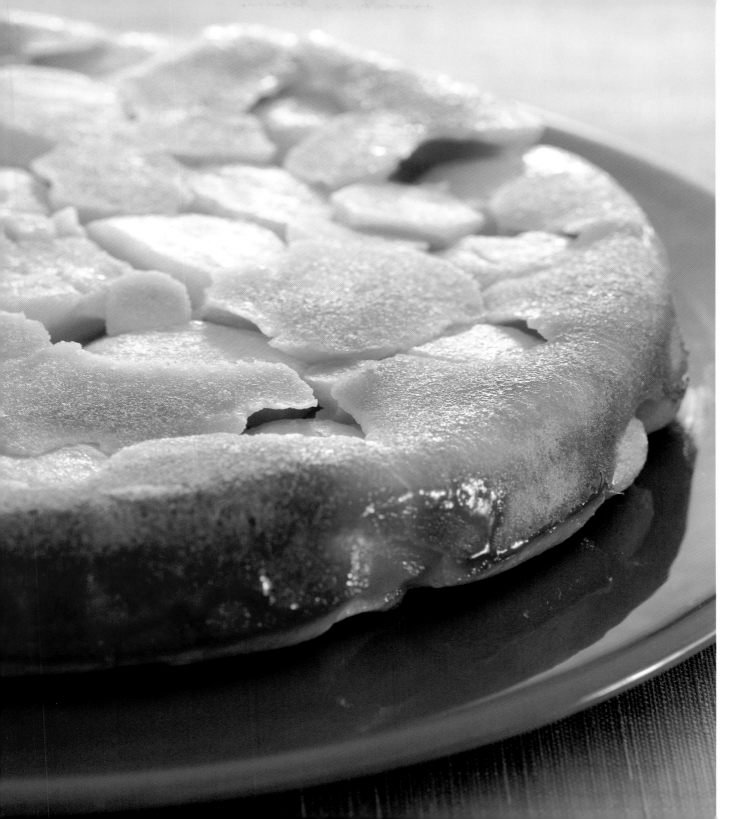

Chocolate Truffles

Makes about 30 truffles

Preparation: 20 minutes

- 6oz (160 g) unsweetened cocoa powder
- 3oz (75 g) fine fructose powder
- 5oz (150 g) butter – unsalted
- 2 egg yolks
- 3oz (80 g) low fat crème fraîche

- Remove the butter from the fridge 4 hours before starting the recipe. Do this to ensure the butter is at room temperature when you start working.
- Put the butter in a basin and work with a wooden spoon until the texture is completely smooth.
- Incorporate first the egg yolks, then the fructose and then the cocoa.
- Continue stirring with a spoon until the mixture is completely mixed and smooth again.
- Add the crème fraîche and continue mixing into a stiff paste. If the mixture is too soft, return to the fridge for an hour to stiffen.
- With a spoon form small balls out of the paste and then roll them in cocoa powder.
- Shape the truffles according to fancy.
- Store in the fridge. Allow 15 minutes before serving, once the truffles have been removed from the fridge.

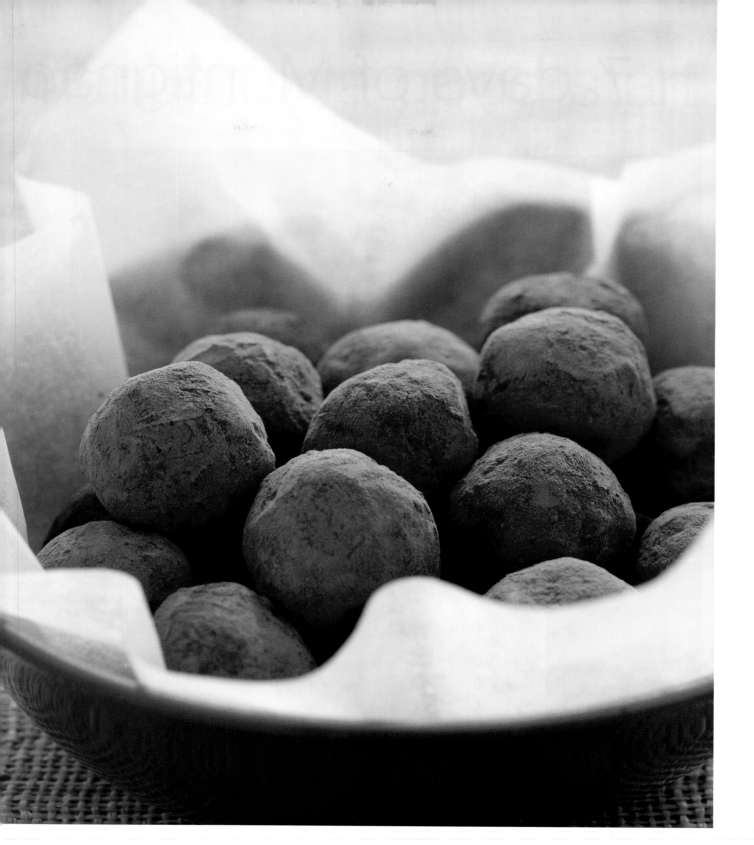